HEMOPHILIA

A Study in Hope and Reality

HEMOPHILIA

A Study in Hope and Reality

By

ALFRED H. KATZ, D.S.W.

Professor, Schools of Public Health and Social Welfare
University of California
Los Angeles, California

CHARLES C THOMAS • PUBLISHER

Springfield · Illinois · U.S.A.

Published and Distributed Throughout the World by

CHARLES C THOMAS • PUBLISHER
Bannerstone House
301-327 East Lawrence Avenue, Springfield, Illinois, U.S.A.
Natchez Plantation House
735 North Atlantic Boulevard, Fort Lauderdale, Florida, U.S.A.

Library of Congress Catalog Card Number: 79-77929

Printed in the United States of America
RV-1

Dedicated to
My Wife and My Daughter

FOREWORD

"Strange it is that our bloods
Of colour, weight and heat, pour'd all together
Would quite confound distinction, yet stand off
In differences so mighty."

All's Well That Ends Well, Act II, Sc.iii

IN this book we propose to discuss mainly the social and psychological problems of hemophilia an hereditary, chronic disorder that affects some sixty thousand persons in the United States. Although hemophilia has been known from antiquity, it has been enshrouded in a veil of popular superstition and fear which has helped prevent its examination in terms of the practical needs of patients and their families We hope in this work to dispel a number of the myths that have surrounded hemophilia in the popular mind and to inform professionals by outlining current understanding of both the physical factors and the social psychological correlates of the disorder.

In order to examine authoritatively the medical aspects of hemophilia the second chapter of the book has been written by a prominent physician who has had extensive clinical experience with hemophiliacs and who is abreast of the current research in this field. The subsequent chapters explore in detail the situation of the hemophiliacs's family, psychological development in the young hemophiliac, the conditions and circumstances surrounding his education and his world of social experience, ranging from the young child's play to adult social relationships in later life. Several chapters based on recent research, will consider in detail the current vocational experience the work limitations and needs of the hemophiliac. Other chapters examine the nature of social and community services necessary to provide the maximum degree of psychosocial normality that the hemophiliac can attain. A final chapter summarizes findings and a comprehensive program of public responsibility for hemophiliacs.

This book is the product of some years of contact with hemophiliacs at firsthand, and in a research capacity. It represents also a conscientious effort to distil the findings from the small but growing number of studies by behavioral scientists, psychiatrists, and others who have recognized that in hemophilia are encapsulated most of the problems of adaptation to chronic illness and social limitation found in other disabling conditions. It is hoped, therefore that the analyses, findings, and conclusions of this study will have applicability beyond the confines of hemophilia.

While the discussions to follow at times will be somewhat technical the intent of this work is to avoid technicalities wherever possible and to describe the circumstances of hemophilic patients in lucid and accessible language. It is the writer's experience that no group is more keenly interested in research and therapeutic developments affecting their immediate welfare than are hemophiliacs and their families and it is therefore to be expected that the latter will constitute an important portion of the readers of this work.

Of at least equal importance to the writer, however, is reaching the various professionals in the community who in one way or another may expect to have some association with the problems of hemophiliacs. Teachers, physicians, nurses, vocational counselors, physical therapists, psychiatrists, psychologists, social workers, and others, it is hoped, will find the present volume useful to them as a summary of current knowledge and a starting point for their helping efforts.

CONTENTS

HEMOPHILIA

A Study in Hope and Reality

Chapter 1

HEMOPHILIA – AN OVERVIEW

HEMOPHILIA, which is as old as recorded history, is the most important of a small group of defects in blood clotting which may be transmitted by inheritance. While estimates of its incidence and prevalence vary, as far as can be judged at the present time, hemophiliacs number about one in every ten thousand of the population, the affected individuals being almost all males. Hemophilia is thus not an exceptionally rare or esoteric condition. Projecting the estimate to the current population, we reach a figure of some twenty to thirty thousand sufferers from well-defined forms of hemophilia in the United States, with perhaps an equally large borderline population of mild bleeders.

In about 40 percent of known cases, there is no recorded history of hemophilia in the ancestry. This can be explained either on the basis of hidden inheritance through generations of female carriers (who do not themselves bleed abnormally) or because of "new" cases that arise from genetic mutation. There is as yet no reliable way of picking out female carriers by laboratory tests. That many, if not most, of the new cases must be the result of mutation is made likely by the fact that hemophilia has not become extinct over many centuries, despite the high mortality in childhood that was unavoidable until recently.

The incidence of hemophilia cuts across social, economic, geographical, and ethnic lines and does not show a specific association to ethnic characteristics as, for example, does another blood disorder, sickle cell anemia, which is confined to members of the Negro race. Among the sufferers from hemophilia all orders of severity are found; the estimate of twenty to thirty thousand cases of classical and well-defined types does not include many mild "bleeders," whose symptoms are of such little severity as to show up only from a serious wound or at the time of surgery or other major body stress.

The social consequences of hemophilia begin to manifest themselves in early childhood and continue throughout the lifetime of the sufferer.

With recent advances in medical science, the life expectancy of hemophiliacs may be approaching that of the general population. Dramatic research advances in the past two decades, resulting in improved methods of transfusion and management make possible surgery and other drastic therapies that have reduced the mortality of hemophiliacs. The high mortality of such patients in earlier years can be inferred from the fact that in a recent study of 1,055 hemophiliacs conducted by the writer, only twenty-seven men aged sixty and over were found. They were 2.6 percent of the group studied as contrasted with the more than 20 percent of the general population who are in this age group. There are many indications that the current generation of young and middle-aged hemophiliacs will survive for far longer average periods than did hemophiliacs of thirty years ago. This lengthening in life expectancy, unless remedial community services are widely offered and utilized, however, could have the effect of increasing the problems of social living for hemophiliacs. As in other fields of chronic illness, advances in medical knowledge and improvements of care have accentuated the need for attention to the psychosocial problems.

Hemophilia and "Social Deviance"

Popular misconceptions abound regarding hemophilia. If his condition is known, the hemophiliac is often regarded with apprehension and fear, and thought to be liable to constant bleeding, and thus incapable of a relatively normal existence. This popular conception of the hemophiliac, which goes against realistic current knowledge and certainly against the hemophiliac's desires, has placed him in a rather special category in society. In short, he is popularly regarded as a social deviant, one who may have difficulty in performing the usual social roles in the socially expected fashion. The hemophiliac may internalize these adverse beliefs that society holds, especially since the coagulation defect can often pose a threat to survival, and a considerable portion of the hemophiliac's life must thus be lived in a framework of ever-present danger.

Whether or not it poses a direct threat to his survival the individual's inheritance of a coagulation defect has wide and distinct social consequences. These may, but do not have to, involve the patient and his family in a web of emotional and social adjustment problems.

The patient's mother, as the female carrier of the defective gene, is not herself clinically affected by it. The father, not himself a sufferer from the disease, is nevertheless a member of a family group in which hemophilia usually imposes manifold problems that can strain and distort family relationships.

The third member of the affected group is, of course, the patient. In the interactions that develop within the family group, many of the influences, attitudes, and directions that will determine the hemophiliac's patterns of social coping and his possibilities of later adaptations are laid down. Other early social relationships—with friends, neighbors, teachers, schoolmates—are also very important.

The ever-present possibilities of physical trauma for the hemophiliac include the unheralded and unpredictable occurrence of internal bleeding, the necessary frequency of transfusions and other medical treatments, and the consequent necessity to have expensive and technically complex medical care available and accessible constantly; the possibility of crippling deformities in the joints resulting in temporary or permanent disability. These and other consequences—not least the economic—mark this as a defect with enormously widespread effects. In these consequences not only the patient but also the whole family is involved. Patterns of child care and rearing, permissiveness, and discipline become, as we shall see, crucial variables in the personality development and adult adaptations of the patient.

Conforming to the expectation that hemophilia in a child will bring a crucial involvement of his entire family, recent studies—which will be discussed in detail at a later point—indicate that there is a close relationship between the patterns of the young child's upbringing and his subsequent adaptation in young adulthood and adult life. For example, data from interviews from the writer's own research suggest that the specific parental pattern of permissiveness and protectiveness is the most important variable that influences the degree of self-direction and independence that the adult hemophiliac develops (13). This finding is now being tested in further studies.

A closely related and highly important idea is that of the self-image of the hemophiliac. Data from the writer's study suggest the conclusion that in relation to employment it is not just the degree of impairment and disability that determines unemployment, under-employment, or total absence from job market. Employment status is almost equally dependent upon the hemophiliac's *self-perception* of himself as either an employable, as a chronically handicapped person, or as something in between. The concept of oneself as employable and relatively autonomous makes it possible for many hemophiliacs, whether or not suffering frequent illness and physical handicap, to function in a comparatively normal manner in work roles and family roles. By contrast, the absence of such a self-concept is associated, even for the moderately or mildly physically handicapped individual, with withdrawal from the job market, apathy, economic dependency, and general resignation to an unproductive existence.

The idea that the self-concept of hemophiliacs is related to attitudes and behavior of the members of the patient's immediate family, of his parents, siblings, and of "significant others" toward him conforms to modern sociopsychological principles Perhaps the best and most thorough presentation of this theoretical framework, in which the family is viewed as the matrix of socialization, is set forth in the work of Parsons and Bales(15). Our own study also suggested that for this condition which affects chiefly males, a masculine figure to identify with is of great significance. Such identification is obtained in the first instance from the hemophiliac's father, but if it is not appropriately available there, other adults and peer groups of friends can become highly significant surrogates.

Thus, we find in hemophilia both an unusual medical problem and a condition having some special characteristics which help to shape the hemophiliac's whole life and destiny. To recapitulate the major points we have discussed are as follows:

1. Hemophilia is sex-linked, being confined almost entirely to males.

2. It is hereditary and always present from birth even though its manifestations may not have been observed until later.

3. It is incurable, in the sense that there is no way at present, known or imaginable, of being able to reverse the genetic defect.

4. It is lifelong. Although hemophiliacs often learn to take care of themselves better so they don't get into difficulty as frequently as they grow older, the defect in the clotting mechanism remains constant.

5. It is a threat to life and hampers normal adjustment, so that it poses great and protracted strains upon family living.

These points will be illuminated further as we consider the nature of the biological and medical problems of hemophilia in the following chapter.

Chapter 2

HEMOPHILIA—MEDICAL ASPECTS

CECIL E. C. HARRIS, M.D., F.R.C.P.*

THERE is a small group of hereditary and congenital defects of blood coagulation of which classical hemophilia is the most common and the most important. Developed only in the past few decades, our present conception of blood clotting is that of a highly complex series of interreactions involving several biologically distinct substances. From a bewildering crop of terminologies, an International Committee on Nomenclature produced order by assigning Roman numerals to clotting factors upon the identity of which there was reasonable agreement. Thirteen such factors are recognized at the present time.

It would serve no useful purpose here to elaborate any detailed schema of the coagulation mechanism, because such would be largely hypothetical and probably confusing. However, for practical purposes hemostasis, or the staunching of blood flow from a wound, may be conceived as occurring in two phases, the first of which involves active blood vessel constriction coupled with the formation of plugs composed of platelet aggregates. The second phase comprises three distinct reactions: the formation of thromboplastin or prothrombinactivator, the conversion of prothrombin to thrombin, and the conversion of fibrinogen to the definitive clotting substance, fibrin. Thus, for descriptive purposes, there are four stages in clotting, each of which may be affected by the congenital absence of an essential clotting factor. It should be noted that some consider the problem to be due to an excess of antagonists rather than a dearth of substance, but this remains controversial. A comprehensive list of congenital defects of

*Dr. Harris is Chief. Hematologist at St. Mary's Hospital in Montreal; Medical Consultant to the Canadian Hemophilia Society, and Chairman of the Medical Advisory Committee, World Federation of Hemophilia.

hemostasis is given in Table I with division into the four stages already defined; von Willebrand's disease is remarkable in that it involves two of the stages.

Classical hemophilia (hemophilia A – factor VIII) and Christmas disease (hemiphilia B – factor IX) differ only in details and together embrace more than 90 percent of all congenital "bleeders"; it is convenient to include both disorders under the title of "hemophilia" for most practical discussions, and this convention will frequently be used in this chapter There exist about four cases of factor VIII deficiency for every case of factor IX deficiency and, on the average, the classical cases tend to be somewhat more severe in their clinical manifestations. The inheritance is sex-linked and recessive, which means that, following mendelian laws, hemophilia is a disease of males; it is transmitted by asymptomatic females, and only by double inheritance can an affected female arise. In all other congenital defects of hemostasis, inheritance is autosomal, dominant in some and recessive in others, so that males and females equally are affected.

It is not possible accurately to determine the incidence of hemophilia, and there are two reasons why our present statistics likely err on the low side. Not all of the severe cases are "found" by or known to the statisticians. There is no clear distinction between mild "bleeders" and "normals"; indeed, there is an appreciable degree of overlapping. In various surveys of different Caucasian populations, however, reports vary from 1:2,000 down to 1:30,000 of the males. In North America (U.S.A. and Canada) the incidence would seem to be 1-2:10,000 of the males.

There is much variation in titer of clotting factors from one individual to another, the range being roughly between 30 percent and 160 percent of the average. Below 30 percent, mild bleeders exist who live normal lives until the defect is made manifest by some injury, commonly dental extractions or surgical interventions. Below 5 percent, apparently spontaneous hemorrhages and hemarthroses occasionally occur; while below 1 percent, abnormal bleeding and frequent involvement of joints usually start in infancy to give the classical picture of hemophilia. The severity of the defect breeds true in any one family while the level in the individual is subject to transient fluctuations associated with stress, exercise, and pregnancy. Clinical severity does not always precisely parallel the laboratory assessment, and psychological factors influencing capillaries may determine the variation.

In sex-linked hemophilia, all the sons of an affected husband married to a normal wife will be normal, while all the daughters will be carriers of the defect. With a carrier wife married to a normal man, there is an even chance for sons to be affected and for daughters to be carriers. It is thus possible for the defect to be passed down through several generations of female carriers without expression in a male until it is forgotten that the problem ever existed. Such hidden inheritance doubtless explains some of the cases without known hemophiliac ancestors, these forming about 40 percent of reported series. Other sufferers without known family history could be the result of mutation, and geneticists consider that a high rate of spontaneous mutation must be invoked to explain the persistence of a defect, recorded in ancient writings, which commonly denied survival of the individual to maturity.

As a consequence of these genetical facts, it must be appreciated that the problem of hemophilia may arise in any family at any time, and thus it is a problem which is of potential concern to all. From the estimates previously given, it follows that approximately one of every 10,000 live male births will be an unanticipated hemophiliac.

With blood component therapy a reality of only the past fifteen years, already the prognosis for survival has been reversed and most sufferers attain adult life. As generation succeeds generation, an increase in prevalence of the problem seems inevitable unless a radical "cure" can be found or unless rigid family planning be adopted. It would obviously be of material help could we distinguish in the laboratory between carrier and noncarrier females, but it is not as yet generally accepted that this can be done with reasonable confidence.

It has been pointed out that mild bleeders become problems only when injured or when subjected to surgery. It is enough to be aware of the possibility, to screen out and identify such cases in the laboratory, and to have available the facilities for managing severe hemophiliacs. Clinical suspicion may be aroused because of abnormal bleeding after circumcision, dental extractions, or tonsillectomy. Bruising may be noticed when the infant starts to crawl and painful swollen knees when he starts to walk. To screen capillary defects the tourniquet and the "bleeding time" tests are available, the latter being very crude. A thromboplastin screening test is used for the second stage of hemostasis and the one-stage prothrombin time for the third. Blood lacking fibrinogen will not clot at all. Should a defect be revealed by these preliminary studies, detailed and somewhat complicated investigations must then be done to identify the factor or factors involved and to assess the severity of the defect.

In hemophilia, the most common problem is that of seemingly spontaneous hemorrhages into various joints, most often the knees, the ankles, the elbows, and the hips. There results exquisite pain, deep and persistent, totally filling awareness and excluding sleep. There is limitation of movement and there may be visible swelling. Untreated, the agony continues for as much as five weeks. Repeated episodes lead to progressive degenerative osteoarthritis, crippling, muscular atrophy, and unstable joints–the seat of chronic arthritic pain.

Unprovoked bleeding into other sites also is frequently encountered. Bruises, subcutaneous accumulations, and hemorrhages into muscles do not often constitute a challenge; although a cyst-like collection of blood may take long to resolve and sufficient tension may be built up in restricted compartments such as those of the forearm and lower leg, as to compress nerves, leading to actual paralysis. So also may retroperitoneal hemorrhage, which usually is associated with the psoas muscle, lead to compression of the lumbar plexus which may proceed to widespread sensory loss and to wasting of the quadriceps with consequent serious crippling.

Internally, bleeding from the kidneys and the small bowel commonly occurs, the former giving hematuria and renal "colic" and the latter a picture of intestinal obstruction. The pain of chronic arthritis leads to the use of analgesics which often contain acetylsalicylic acid, which may cause a form of hemorrhagic gastritis with any degree of bleeding from occult, leading to iron-depletion anemia, to massive and exsanguinating. Peptic ulceration does not seem to be any more frequent in hemophiliacs despite the anxieties of their condition, but fleeting tranquillity through alcohol may repeatedly be sought with ultimate cirrhosis as the price, especially if there has also been an episode of serum hepatitis to damage the liver.

Epistaxis is another common problem which, if not associated with trauma, may stem from the want of an effective humidifier in a centrally heated home. As with nosebleeds, so with all of the manifestations described, hemorrhage may be provoked by an injury, albeit trivial—a twist, a strain, a fall, a blow, an injection, petty challenges which nonetheless may create a major problem. Whether or not this happens may depend upon the curious and unexplained fact that, without detectable change in laboratory findings, the hemophiliac sometimes may indulge with impunity in vigorous activities while at other times turning over in bed is a risk.

Increasingly there is concern over the effects of a blow to the head. Intracranial hemorrhage seems to be more often a cause of death than in the past, perhaps because of the reduction in mortality from other crises in the life of a bleeder. After a deceptive latent period the signs of subdural or subarachnoid hemorrhage may arise following, for example, an automobile accident. Less blatant injuries may give rise to petechial hemorrhages which are invoked to explain the increased incidence of epilepsy reported in some series.

Contrary to popular opinion, ordinary cuts and lacerations seldom pose much of a problem once a few basic "tricks" are acquired, but dental extractions and the removal of tonsils involving the tearing of tissues, invariable result in copious and sustained bleeding. On the other hand, "clean" surgical incisions usually may be readily controlled. Thus it is that a history of unusual blood loss starting a few hours after the removal of a tooth may be of particular significance in suggesting the presence of mild hemophilia even if other inquiries yield negative or equivocal results.

The long-term effect of severe hemophilia is, above all, manifest in the limb joints, of which the knees are the most important.

Repeated hemorrhages produce in sequence synovial thickening, fibrosis, erosion of cartilage, subchondral cysts, irregularity of growth, and perhaps fibrous ankylosis. Muscle wasting and osteoporosis are accompaniments. There is evidence that prompt and effective treatment of each episode of acute hemarthrosis prevents, minimizes, or retards joint damage of this nature; such an approach makes imperative the provision of special facilities in any hospital undertaking the care of hemophiliacs.

This brings us to the point of specifying the particular provisions desirable for optimal management of hemophilia. The key figure in most instances is a clinical hematologist who has developed an interest in the field and who is capable of appreciating the overall picture–medical, paramedical, and socioeconomic. The team must include exponents of physical medicine, of orthopedics, of general surgery, of psychiatry, and of dentistry, with yet others as occasion may demand. The entire staff must be imbued with a sense of urgency as to the promptness with which treatment of each episode should be initiated, an attitude sometimes difficult to sustain in the face of demands by other patients, especially as the hemophiliac turns up so frequently that familiarity may dull the edge of sympathy. Nursing supervisors and charge nurses are indispensable allies in maintaining the efficiency of the program.

The first line of defense is the emergency department or some other area in which transfusions may be given on an outpatient basis for episodes of acute hemarthrosis. Delay caused by paper work, by the absence of someone to start the infusion, or by any other avoidable factor cannot be tolerated; adequate facilities and careful planning are required. The laboratory beforehand will have had to identify the clotting defect, and this is not an examination that can be done at a moment's notice. The blood bank must be kept well stocked with plasma components which may the more readily be achieved as community blood-bank systems expand and increase in efficiency; the advent of multiple-unit plastic packs for blood collection permits the provision of several components from each donation, thus limiting the need for additional donors. The trend is toward the production of concentrated preparations of the various clotting factors, and we may therefore anticipate treatment by intravenous injection of a syringeful of potent material rather than by transfusions of unmodified plasma. This will facilitate outpatient management, provided that the sense of urgency not be diminished.

The same background resources are, of course, ready to deal with the patient who has to be admitted, whether this be because of hemarthrosis too severe to be handled in the outpatient unit or because of any of the myriad other manifestations of abnormal bleeding. Particular mention must be made of the fact that the pain of hemarthrosis is severe and sustained; the individual has had many such crises in the past and he anticipates many more in the future. It can be appreciated that tolerance to pain is impaired and substantial dosage of painkillers often has to be used, raising the bogey of addiction which, however, rarely becomes a real problem, provided that narcotics are used only for acute hemarthrosis and not for chronic hemarthropathy.

The experienced team will go on to tackle elective procedures with confidence, and only the specter of the refractory state remains so far insuperable. Dental extractions, appendectomy and, indeed, the whole range of abdominal surgical procedures can be and have been done. Of course, hemostatic control by component administration is needed until healing is complete, and this requires the support of a major blood-bank program.

The future lies in the application of these principles from earliest childhood onward, with regular prophylactic injections for severe cases suffering frequent hemarthroses. Only in this way can we hope to lessen or to prevent the crippling which typical hemophiliacs sustain in their formative years and which handicaps them throughout their life.

It has been possible to present no more than a digest of technical and clinical matter relating to hemophilia. For further information and for reference, the following publications are recommended.

TABLE I

Stage 1.	Von Willebrand's disease Hereditary telangiectasia Ehlers-Danlos syndrome
Stage 2.	Factor VIII (hemophilia A) Factor IX (hemophilia B) Factor XI (PTA deficiency) Von Willebrand's disease
Stage 3.	Prothrombin (factor II) Factor VII Factor V Factor X
Stage 4.	Fibrinogen (factor I) Fibrin-stabilizing factor (factor XIII)

Chapter 3

PERSONAL AND SOCIAL CHARACTERISTICS OF HEMOPHILIACS

WHO is affected by hemophilia and what kind of people are they?

We have already indicated that the general incidence of hemophilia is about one per ten thousand males in any given population. This rate holds true for the United States and Canada; for Australia, Holland, and Sweden—all countries where there is relatively good statistical reporting of health problems. The rate is reported as being between two and five per ten thousand males in Switzerland, where church records dating back several centuries confirm the existence of a highly stable, highly inbred population in some of the isolated mountain cantons. Presumably, over the centuries, concentration of the genetic pool has resulted in a higher number of hemophiliacs proportionate to the population there than elsewhere.

Since most studies of hemophiliacs are on clinical treatment methods or blood coagulation, and usually report on only a small number of cases, there is not much information on the general social characteristics of the hemophilic population. Our own study, conducted between 1962 and 1964 is probably the largest and most comprehensive one that has been made(13). This study did not attempt to look at all hemophiliacs, children and adults, but rather secured information on hemophiliacs sixteen years and older.

A total of 1055 men were included in the study, living in all parts of the United States, and of all conditions of health and social circumstances. The findings of our study illustrate some of the social characteristics of the adult hemophiliac population and permit the following generalizations to be made.

Most Hemophiliacs Now Survive Into at Least Middle Age

The hemophilia population at present primarily is composed of the young and middle-aged.

Owing to the life-threatening nature of the disease, until a period of approximately twenty years ago it was rare for a severely affected hemophiliac to survive into late middle age or old age. Our data on age distribution reflect this fact.

TABLE II

AGE DISTRIBUTION OF 1,055 HEMOPHILIACS OVER SIXTEEN

Years	*Number*	*Percent*	*Years*	*Percent*
16-19	237	22.5	under 30	56
20-29	357	33.8	under 40	78
30-39	231	21.9	under 50	91
40-49	132	12.5		
50-59	68	6.4		
60-69	22	2.1		
70-79	5	.5		
No information	3	.3		
	1,055	100.0		

Based on medical advances, a change can be projected for the future, with the current middle-aged group surviving in a larger proportion than in the previous generation, and the young approximating the life expectancy of the nonhandicapped population. The implications of this change for all programs of care are profound.

Hemophilia Is Not Specific to Any Race, Ethnic or Socioeconomic Group

From our study, from clinical observations and from the known patterns of genetic transmission, it seems reasonable to conclude that hemophiliacs include persons from all walks of life.

Although the illness is genetically determined, there are no findings indicating that particular races or ethnic strains have a larger incidence, as for example, in the association of sickle cell anemia with the Negro race. In our study, 90.4 percent were Caucasian, 3.4 percent Negro, .5 percent Orientals; while 3.5 percent checked "other" without further explanation. The non-Caucasian population in the United States is probably underrepresented in the sample; this may be attributed to cultural factors, probable underrepresentation in the hemophilia associations, and lower accessibility to medical facilities.

Other than race, we did not obtain data on ethnic backgrounds of our respondents, but from surnames it seemed to include persons of Anglo-Saxon, Middle European, Scandinavian, Jewish, Greek, Armenian, Japanese, and other ethnic groups. There also seems to be no geographic specificity in the incidence of the disease. While a larger concentration of hemophiliacs was to be found living in the big cities of the East and West coasts, this fact can be accounted for by the presence in these locations of specialized treatment facilities.

Many Hemophiliacs Marry and Have Children

This population, afflicted with a chronic and often severely disabling condition, in which the pattern of genetic transmission is clearly understood and realized by most sufferers, nevertheless marry and have children in a substantial proportion. Table III indicates the proportion of married, single, divorced, or separated individuals in our study.

TABLE III

MARITAL STATUS OF 1,055 HEMOPHILIACS

Marital Status	*Number*	*Percent*
Single	538	51.0
Married	486	46.1
Divorced	19	1.8
Separated	4	.4
Widowed	6	.6
No information	2	.2
	1,055	100.1

It is also of interest to note the number of children in hemophiliac families. About 30 percent of the married couples are childless. The number of children reported in the others is shown in Table IV.

TABLE IV

NUMBER OF CHILDREN OF 1,055 HEMOPHILIACS

Number of Children	*Number of Respondents*	*Percent*
None	661	62.65
1	129	12.23
2	142	13.46
3	70	6.64
4	36	3.41
5+	16	1.52
	1,055	99.91

It has been estimated that up to 40 percent of hemophiliacs cannot trace their condition in their family history(9). In some instances the disease has remained hidden for at least seven generations. An unknown number have hemophilia as a result of spontaneous gene mutation. While about 45 percent in our study stated they had no known hemophiliac relatives this cannot be taken as an accurate reflection of the incidence of inheritance versus gene mutation in the sample, since there may have been inadequate family records, concealment of the disease, and incomplete questionnaire responses.

Most Hemophiliacs Live with Families

The number of hemophiliacs who live alone is quite small (4.8 percent). Table V shows the living arrangements that were reported by our respondents.

The implications of living alone could be quite serious for sufferers from hemophilia. During periods of hemorrhage, there frequently has to be bed rest; there is a frequent necessity for transfusions or other medical care. Emergency transfusions by a

TABLE V

LIVING ARRANGEMENTS, 1,055 HEMOPHILIACS

	Number	*Percent*
Alone	51	4.83
Parents	461	43.70
Wife	149	14.12
Wife and children	320	30.33
Wife and own or wife's parents	16	1.52
Other relatives (sister, aunt)	34	3.22
Other (hospital, rooming house)	30	2.84
No information	4	.38
	1,055	100.93

doctor who comes to the home have been frequent episodes in the life of hemophiliacs. Solitary living would magnify the physical adjustment problems of the hemophiliac and in some cases might reduce his overall chances for physical survival in case of difficulty.

The Educational Status of Hemophiliacs Is a Mixed Picture

Of the 1,055 hemophiliacs in our study, 279 were still in school, most in their late teens and twenties. Including this group, a broad range of school achievement was found, from some who had no formal education at all, to some who had completed graduate school with a Ph.D., M.D., M.A., M.S. degree or teaching credentials. Table VI gives the distribution for highest grade achieved.

Table VI shows that 34 percent did not complete high school and probably many of those in the "No information" category did not finish or even attend high school. *Twenty-three percent received education beyond the high school level.*

About 65 percent of the entire sample attended regular elementary schools, and 14 percent went to regular elementary school in addition to attendance at special schools and/or tutoring. Six percent indicated they had received no elementary school education other than private tutoring, either by a board of education home tutor or a private tutor.

TABLE VI

HIGHEST GRADE COMPLETED: 1,055 HEMOPHILIACS

Highest Grade	*Still in School*	*Out of School*
6th grade and under	1	55
7th through 9th	23	120
10th through 11th	49	91
12th or graduated from high school	51	206
Freshman, college	15	34
Sophomore, college	21	43
Junior, college	11	15
Senior or college graduate	12	44
Some graduate school	10	12
Completed graduate school with degree	5	33
No information	81	123
	279	776

Sixty percent of the total were attending or had attended regular high school; and 4 percent, regular high school in addition to trade school. Only 8 percent indicated they had received tutoring in addition to high school attendance, and 5 percent had received no high school education other than tutoring.

Many Hemophiliacs Can and Do Work Steadily

Table VII characterizes the employment status of the respondents at the time of the survey (1963-4).

Thus the overall picture we found is that, by and large, the individual hemophiliac had been able to find comparatively steady employment; although the type of employment and level of income is often below what it might have been if he were unhandicapped. As the later chapters on employment will document, the hemophiliac is frequently at a competitive disadvantage in employment and receives a lesser position and salary.

TABLE VII

EMPLOYMENT STATUS: 1,055 HEMOPHILIACS

	Number	*Percent*
Currently employed	552	52.32
Currently unemployed	152	14.41
Retired	12	1.14
Still in school	279	26.45
Never employed	60	5.69
	1,055	100.01

Many Hemophiliacs Have Active Personal and Social Lives

Hemophiliacs who assume more active and independent roles frequently have a well-rounded personal life. They may participate in the Hemophilia Foundation or other form of self-help group. Some 78 percent of the respondents indicated membership in a hemophilia association; 10 percent were not members; 12 percent did not answer the question.

TABLE VIII

TYPES OF LEISURE-TIME ACTIVITIES: 946 HEMOPHILIACS

Type	*Number*	*Percent*
Solitary—e.g. radio and T.V. repair, gardening, electronics, reading	233	24.6
Predominantly solitary—e.g. car repair, playing musical instruments, photography	194	20.5
Mixed—e.g. fishing, hunting, traveling (mixed activities) or fishing and photography, bowling and reading (mixed responses)	280	29.6
Predominance of group activity with some solitary	141	14.9
Group activities—no solitary listed, e.g. dating, visiting, clubs, pool, tennis, table games	98	10.4
	946	100.0

Our findings on this point, to be discussed in detail later, run counter to the popular and often erroneous picture of the hemophiliac as a fragile, sedentary, and socially withdrawn person. It is an old belief that hemophiliacs should be "wrapped in cotton" and kept in an inactive state. Despite many pressures on them in that direction from parents and others, our study indicates that most of the men engage in moderate to very active leisure-time activities.

Table VIII briefly summarizes these findings.

SUMMARY

This chapter has presented some findings of a study regarding the personal and social characteristics of hemophiliacs.

Affecting males almost exclusively, hemophilia is found in persons of all walks of life, and its incidence is not concentrated in any racial, ethnic, or subcultural grouping. It is present at birth, but in clinically mild cases may not be diagnosed until childhood or later. It is a familial disease, and many hemophiliacs have male maternal relatives who are also sufferers.

In the immediate past, many hemophiliacs did not survive, but with medical advances, survival into middle and old age is predictable for most hemophiliacs. Many hemophiliacs marry, have children, are steadily employed, and function in independent social roles.

Some hemophiliacs are chronically disabled in the sociopsychological sense, whatever the nature of their physical condition. These persons are dependent materially and socially and present problems to themselves, their families, and society. Special efforts at rehabilitation should be directed toward them.

A broad range of educational achievement was found from respondents with no formal education to those who have completed university work and advanced degrees. A high percentage of the men, however, were low educational achievers who did not complete high school. The educational level achieved bears a direct relationship to occupational and personal adjustment.

Many hemophiliacs participate in active and even possibly

hazardous leisure-time activities. Thus our data indicate that hemophiliacs desire and are capable of a higher activity level than is generally assumed.

Chapter 4

THE HEMOPHILIAC'S FAMILY: A TOTAL INVOLVEMENT

THE PARENT'S DILEMMA

IN recent years there has been an enormous change in attitudes toward the physically disabled. This change has probably been brought about by several interacting factors: first, the effects of progress in medical science, which has led to notable advances in the treatment, rehabilitation, and prevention of many chronic conditions. Secondly, the "therapeutic optimism" or sense of hope that arises from many previously disabling conditions having been conquered, and which leads to greater energy and effort being devoted to patients previously thought untreatable. And third, from these developments there has come a growing enlightenment of both the public and professionals, a spirit that since something can be done, it is a social and professional obligation to provide the best services and research, to overcome the still unsolved problems.

Yet, these hopeful changes of recent years do not alter the immediate impact that having a handicapped child makes on the parents and families. Each family unit must still struggle to come to terms with the practical and emotional problems that arise when a child is born with some physical and mental defect and who requires special care throughout childhood and perhaps all his life.

Many studies of parents of different categories of chronically handicapped children–the deaf, the blind, cerebral palsied, mentally retarded, asthmatic, diabetic, and other groups of chronically ill children–show that caring for and rearing them presents complex and difficult problems for their parents.

Each disability has some particular characteristics of its own, and each requires some special understanding and some special care. Yet the broad generalization can be made that having a physically or mentally handicapped child tends to set off parents into a group with heightened problems of social adjustment and living.

While being parents of a handicapped child is generally difficult, being parents of a hemophiliac child presents some singular problems. When her child has been diagnosed as a hemophiliac, the mother must first deal with the problems of heredity. She comes to realize that she has unwittingly transmitted a defective gene to her son, which results in a lifelong impairment of coagulation. If there was a known family history, that is, if a father, grandfather, brother, or uncle of the mother was a known hemophiliac, it is natural for her to experience a mixture of guilt, fear, and apprehension about the future: emotions that may be so strong as to immobilize her. Especially frequent, where there is a known family history, is guilt or self-blame; for the parents realize they have gambled with the known odds of heredity—and have lost. But as the "female carrier" the mother may feel particularly responsible and the father may blame her too, consciously or unconsciously. A marriage that is not securely founded can be sorely stressed by these emotional trauma in the first months after diagnosis of hemophilia has been established. If there is no prior knowledge of a hereditary background of hemophilia, the situation of the mother may arouse less guilt and less strain on the marital relationship, but the other elements in the parents' emotional distress are present. It is, after all, a norm in our competitive society that every woman gives birth to a beautiful, whole, perfect child—the charming infant of the baby-food commercials. Deviation from this norm, from the expectations of society—that is, of relatives, neighbors, friends—is immediately damaging and threatening to both parents' egos, their individual and collective self-images. To produce a deviant or defective child is somehow to have failed in one of the great tests of social status—that of parenthood.

The parents of the newly diagnosed sufferer from hemophilia

face not only these often profound psychological and social upsets, but they also have a deep, many-sided, and continuing "reality problem" as well. Care for a hemophiliac youngster requires constant watchful vigilance. Attention must be given to the ever-present possibilities of physical harm—the infant can roll over, bruise himself against a corner, cut himself on a sharp edge or a toy, or take a toddler's slight fall. The external or internal bleeding that results from these everyday occurrences, or the more serious bleeding into a joint or organ—all can occur easily, sometimes spontaneously, and all require prompt medical attention. The inexperienced parent can be alarmed at the first bleeding that goes on too long or at hematomas that take too long to disappear. While the child is too young to speak, he cannot make known his needs or where he is hurting, but may show his discomfort in irritability or listlessness.

As the child gets older, reaching the stages of crawling, standing, walking—as he explores his environment, which is part of the normal drive of every developing organism—the parents' problem grows. They now face a psychological "uncertainty" problem. They are told that normal psychological and social growth requires that their child be encouraged to explore his world as fully as possible, yet they are checked by the knowledge that unless the child is protected from physical hazards, serious damage may result.

Thus, for hemophiliacs' parents, the crucial and pervasive dilemma arises: to permit or to restrict? Out of this dilemma comes the key problem in the rearing of a hemophiliac child: treading the narrow line between *necessary physical protectiveness* and *overprotection*—trading known physical risks for unknown psychological hazards.

A series of research studies have quite clearly demonstrated that the way this dilemma is resolved strongly affects the kind of personality the hemophiliac acquires and strongly influences his adjustment in later life.

In the writer's study, it was found that the lesser risks were the physical ones; that overprotectiveness can lead to psychological crippling, to the creation of "drop-out" personalities, of hemophiliacs who see themselves as "handicapped," as "different"; who are underachievers in their social adjustment, in work, in family life, in social participation.

This is how our study characterized this group of hemophiliacs—a minority, it is true, but one having strong and definite characteristics:

> We consider this group of hemophiliacs to be sociopsychologically disabled. From a psychological viewpoint they can be characterized as never having established an identity or self-concept as a socially competent and productive individual who happens to have the limiting condition of hemophilia. Rather, the self-concept is that of a chronically handicapped person and, therefore, a social deviant. The affliction, with hemophilia and possible related handicaps, is self-perceived as rendering it impossible to carry out normal social expectations. These hemophiliacs are therefore both materially and psychologically dependent on others for sustenance.
>
> This group of "dependent" or "borderline dependent" individuals are a serious problem to themselves, their families, and society. The economic dependency may take the form of their never having worked or received earned income. They may maintain themselves on some form of public assistance, or they may simply be noncontributing members of a household that does not require their financial participation. These individuals do not actively seek employment; if they had some training or employable skills, they have nevertheless withdrawn from the labor market, and believe that they are too severely disabled physically to compete with the nonhandicapped.
>
> Such individuals frequently also have limited social participation and do not contemplate marriage and parenthood; their social interactions are largely limited to members of their immediate family. They do not typically interact or identify with a group of peers or other friends.
>
> If married, these individuals may be supported by the employment of their wives in reversal of the usual household roles, with the wife assuming the economic support of the family and the hemophiliac some household responsibilities. For the single individual who has such character patterns and social roles, and who lives with parents and relatives, anxiety is frequently present among both the parents and the hemophiliac regarding his future after the demise of the parents or potentially caretaking relatives(11).

FACTORS IN THE HEMOPHILIAC'S DEVELOPMENT

Agle and Mattson have shown in a series of studies (1) that the psychological adjustment of hemophiliacs may take several distinct forms. One is compensatory intellectual effort and activity. If physical play must be limited because of actual physical disability, parental cautions, or lack of playmates, hemophilic boys who are thrown on their own resources will read more, watch television, develop quiet hobbies such as stamp or coin collecting, learn a musical instrument, become proficient in an unusual field of knowledge. Such compensatory behavior, of course, can occur in many other situations; for a hemophiliac, it can help him cope with his enforced periods at rest in home or in hospital.

Probably this factor has given rise to the impression of many parents that their hemophilic sons are of superior intellectual ability. While some, of course, are (one could compile a "Who's Who" of distinguished people in various fields who were or are hemophilic), there is no evidence to suggest that hemophiliacs have other than the usual distribution of average, above-average and below-average intellectual abilities.

With hemophiliacs, as with the physically or socially handicapped in general, the trick is to ensure that they have the chance to develop the maximum use of capacities they possess.

Opportunity in a technological society is closely linked to education. And here, as we shall have occasion to see, the hemophiliac is often disadvantaged, despite the compensatory activity and effort we have noted.

Disadvantage can result from long-enforced school absences, from no or poor academic and vocational counseling, from a kind of discrimination in higher education which makes it harder for a physically handicapped individual to gain access to, to keep up with, and to complete a college or graduate school.

While society's attitudes are gradually changing, they may not change fast enough to benefit the individual hemophiliac who may live in a particular area which has not changed with the times. It is not easy for a hemophiliac to uproot himself and move to an area where educational opportunities are greater, since often the first imperative is to stay close to a reliable source of medical care. The relationship of the hemophiliac to his doctor or treatment center, as well as to his source of blood supply, is frequently a close one—one that is not lightly exchanged for a better school somewhere else.

Another common psychological reaction found in the hemophiliac is a tendency toward risk-taking behavior. This is dare-devil or defiant behavior, of the kind that is often associated with physically normal adolescents.

Alby and Coen, Agle and Mattson, and other researchers have associated such risk-taking behavior with the more extreme forms of overprotection by parents. A hemophilic boy who feels unduly and unrealistically limited in his activities because of parental fears may break out of parental restrictions explosively. He may engage in the very activities his parents fear most. For example, one of the subjects in our own study was a dare-devil motorcycle racer, who had had several narrow squeaks, but had so far escaped serious injury. He had started racing at age sixteen, unknown to his parents, and when they forbade further such pursuits, he left home and become a "circuit rider" competitor. Psychologists in this interpretation have also speculated that such behavior contains an element of magical "denial"—the hemophiliac seeks to prove his invulnerability by frequently exposing himself to danger.

Still another type of reaction is passivity, as described in the opening chapter. Here, the hemophiliac perceives the protective attitudes and fears of his parents and others in his environment and internalizes them to the extent that he comes to regard himself as incapable of the usual activities of a boy and a man. He relies on others to meet his physical needs and gradually withdraws from a world that he perceives as full of menace. Not all the perceived menaces are physical and material; the passive-dependent hemophiliac also comes to fear social contacts, competition, the ordinary give-and-take of life in competitive and social situations—school, the play group, a job. Such hemophiliacs—and it should be stressed they constitute a minority—become "dropouts"; they withdraw from life but continue to resent their dependency and passivity and what they are missing as they grow older. And they present a serious problem as well for those who love and care for them, since dependency engenders resentment on both sides—in those who exhibit it and in those who must cater to it.

Contrasted with these forms of *unhealthy* reaction are the responses to hemophilia that we can term realistic. Here, the appropriate limitations set by hemophilia are observed, but the direction is toward aiding and creating a constructive personal adjustment—living within the limitations of hemophilia, but living actively, not merely existing passively, and exercising all the physical and mental muscles and capacities.

In our study, we asked adult hemophiliacs, "What advice would you give the parents of a hemophiliac?" In an overwhelming majority, the answer was to encourage activity, experimentation, and social contacts; not to keep the boy at home under observation twenty-four hours a day, but to encourage his play to the maximum, even risking physical trauma in the interests of the growth of his independence and self-confidence. Body-contact sports like football should be avoided; but there is a wide area of physical activity—from swimming through tennis—that can be engaged in. But, further, a normal or realistic response encourages the development of social contacts and the growth of many compensatory intellectual skills. Where the hemophilic boy is encouraged to try, to test out his dormant capacities, to interact, and even to compete with others, the foundations of an adjusted personality are laid. We shall have more to say about the self-concept later; here, it is enough to mention that if, as seems reasonable, a goal of our efforts is the inculcation and development of social competence and a positive self-image, the two are mutually dependent and reinforce each other. A healthy self-image results at least partly from the acceptance, stimulation, and esteem of others. Social competence describes success in carrying out tasks and goals that society puts forward. So both become an aim for the hemophiliac.

THE MOTHERS OF HEMOPHILIACS

These points bring us to a further consideration of the hemophiliac's family—his parents and siblings.

Agle, Mattson, and Gross have studied a number of mothers of hemophiliacs in an attempt to seek the widest possible understanding of their reactions and of technics for counseling with parents.

One of the components of an adaptive use of reality is the use of some common defense mechanisms, among them temporary withdrawal and denial. Mattson and Gross state that

> serious hemorrhagic episodes in the younger boys, three to eight years old, often resulted in a withdrawal type of reaction, with a minimal interest in the environment. Severe pain, in connection with immobilizing medical procedures and a certain apprehensive alertness on the part of the staff seemed to be associated with this transient withdrawal response. As soon as the physical distress subsided, the boys quickly resumed their verbal and affective interaction with the parents and the ward personnel. The reappearance of the patents' use of denial always accompanied this behavioral change. The previous painful sensations and the still present discomfort were minimized or denied, and the boys' attention turned toward the discharge date and return to school. Denial, as well as isolation of feelings associated with hemophilia, was observed in all effectively coping patients, from age three years and on, and disappeared temporarily only during some hemorrhagic crises. This persistent use of denial of current discomfort and anticipated future bleeding enabled the boys to maintain hope for a rapid recovery at times of bleeding, for clinical improvement as they grew older, and for more effective medical care. The common fantasy gratifications of the wish for a normal and active life were also made possible through their reliance on denial; an illustration was provided by a nine-year-old bleeder, who told the story about a thrilling dodgem-car race with his hemophilic brother, while he was receiving plasma infusions and had traction applied to his leg.

In their continuing study Mattson and Gross observed both parents and hemophiliacs. They found that

> eight of the thirty-five hemophiliacs showed a prolonged poor adjustment to their illness, and often also poor peer relations and motivation to achieve in school. They seemed to belong to two groups of extremes of behavioral response. One group of boys (3) displayed a strong reluctance to participate in any physical activities with other children because of fears of trauma. They preferred to sit or lie on their beds, reading and watching television, even during symptom-free periods. They passively accepted most treatment procedures and tended to remain depressed and whiny long after a hemorrhagic episode had subsided. Their clinical picture was reminiscent of a beginning passive-dependent state in that these boys were emotionally very close to their constantly worried and overprotective mothers. The other group of bleeders (5), also raised by overanxious mothers, had rebelled against the parental restrictions. They had turned into

very active and daring boys who often incurred trauma and bleeding as a result of their careless participation in body contact sports(14).

This study reemphasizes the point from our own earlier research that realistic-permissive behavior on the part of parents, especially mothers, led to the best outcome for hemophiliac boys.

But what of the mothers themselves? Here, recent research again verifies the common-sense observations or intuitions found in early descriptive writings (e.g. Katz, 1959).

Mattson and Gross state that of the hemophiliacs they studied

most of the mothers of the eight poorly adapted bleeders had shown markedly anxious and restrictive attitudes in raising their hemophilic children. Their overprotective tendencies were often coupled with a strong resentment of their fate. Five of these mothers had witnessed earlier fatal outcomes of hemophilia or other congenital illnesses in their siblings or their own children. They vividly recalled their ensuing persistent fears, sadness, and guilt. Their guilt feelings were further heightened by their cognizance of their genetic responsibility for the transmission of hemophilia.

THE ROLE OF THE FATHER

As to the role of fathers, our earlier research (Katz and Goldy, 1963) pointed to a rather crucial need for the growing hemophiliac to have a masculine model, for identification. Such a father would encourage his son in life activities, including physical play. We felt that fathers who failed to do so, or who joined in a mutual parental overprotection, contributed toward the creation of passive-dependent personalities or conversely sparked the kind of resentment that underlies self-destructive risk-taking.

Mattson and Gross's research confirms this view, since they found that

the fathers of the well-adjusted patients had taken a decisive, active part in caring for their ill sons . . . and provided good masculine models for them. The fathers of the poorly adjusted bleeders had either been absent for several years due to divorce . . . or they had left all initiative and decisions regarding the children to their usually oversolicitous wives.

Mattson and Gross's point that some fathers of hemophiliacs absent themselves from involvement, retreating into work or other activities outside the home, is echoed by the clinical impressions of many physicians and by other research studies. Thus, Bahnson and associates (18), in a recent in-depth psychological study of twenty-two hemophilic boys and young men, report that their fathers were frequently "uninvolved, distant, and cold."

These clinical impressions and research findings about the important paternal role should not be surprising since they accord with common-sense intuitions and psychological theory.

Freudian psychoanalysts have perhaps overemphasized the sexual-competitive aspects of the relationship between the father and the growing boy. Much less emphasized has been the function of the father in opening up the world of social experience and providing a role-model for his son. But in these aspects the father is vital in the formation of the child's character from early infancy.

Forrest has expressed this well:

> The father is the first stranger, the first representative of the outside world. As such, he is uniquely equipped to help the child relate to objective world, to bridge the gap between himself and others. The father can penetrate into the child's private world and lead him out of it. The mother and child bound together in the mutual satisfaction of giving and receiving, live nevertheless in the world of the father.(5).

Pertinent to the hemophilic boy-often subject to physical restrictions-is the father's role in stimulating play and physical activity.

> The value of the play experience, specifically with father, lies in the strong friendly hand offered by the outside world, that can lead the child to important discoveries about himself and the world about him. The sensation of father's strength and responsive experience of his own strength, is the infant's first intimation of the exciting pleasure of nonprotective but stimulating evocative physical contact. It is also his first knowledge that father's strength is available when his own fails. With father, he finds joy in active physical mastery(6).

Particularly important for a child with a physical handicap, the father can offer experiences to the growing boy to help educate him to a realistic perception of himself and the world, to develop the skills needed to deal with the broader society.

Every child has aggressive energies, and with the help of the father these can be properly channeled. The physical skills the boy develops can release his physical energy and enhance his self-esteem by mastery of himself and his environment.

It is also an important role of the father to help the boy discipline his impulses by making definite demands for acceptable behavior by setting clear limits. As Forrest states "Father's own firm demands for acceptable behavior and his ability to tolerate the ensuing frustration and hostility is a necessary support and model"(7).

As the boy grows he is (ideally) included in his father's masculine interests and responsibilities. Not only does the boy develop a taste for and pleasure in activities and values that are appropriately masculine, but also the father's social contributions, his activities in the household and at work become models and examples. The father's inclusion of his son in the chores, problems and work of the home affords the boy experience in learning the thinking, skills, effort, and discipline needed to do a job or solve a problem. He becomes interested in the potential contribution he can make to the welfare of his group, and gains a realistic perception of work as a necessary and natural function of males.

By adolescence, as Forrest writes, "The child must consolidate and define who he is and where he comes from, in preparation for his venture . . . into life in the impersonal social group. He must clarify and integrate his general concepts of himself, of others, and of how to relate to them"(8).

"SPONTANEOUS" BLEEDING AND EMOTIONAL STATES

An aspect of hemophilia that has fascinated several observers is the relationship of emotional tension to the occurrence of hemorrhaging. Poinsard, a psychiatrist, was the first to point out and to study this phenomenon systematically; although it had been mentioned earlier by clinicians and by hemophiliacs themselves. Rasputin's influence on Tsar Nicholas and his wife was reputed to lie in his ability to control through hypnosis the young hemophilic crown prince's bleeding.

In studies by Browne, Agle and Mattson, and the present writer, there are reports either that hemorrhages are particularly likely to occur in times of tension or fear or that hemophiliacs occasionally can induce internal bleeding either as an attention-getting device or as a kind of self-punishment from the guilt of misdeeds such as not following parent's instructions.

Poinsard and his associates have studied the possible connections between emotional states and bleeding, and other investigators are seeking to demonstrate the actual physiological mechanisms involved. In their studies, Poinsard and Bahnson and associates have found that "hemorrhages often were 'spontaneous' and were related to (separation) anxiety or aggressive excitement. Frequently, hemorrhages took place in anticipation of threatening events"(18).

In their previously cited study of hemophilic children, Mattson and Gross found that increased bleeding was preceded by changes in patients' moods so that the children became more "whiny," defiant, and aggressive.

Bahnson and colleagues, extending the studies of Poinsard, found, more specifically, that

> . . . hemorrhages occur when patients feel trapped with the ambivalently perceived mother figure or when actual or symbolic separation from her is impending. A mixture of rage and desire to escape from, and nostalgic and dependent longings for the mother were present in virtually all episodes of spontaneous bleeding into the joints or soft tissues of our patients(2).

It is appropriate and timely that further research to test these ideas and relationships is in progress.

A possibly related fact is that, although the coagulation defect itself does not change over time, many hemophiliacs have reported that as they grow older they have fewer hemorrhages. This common observation may arise from two factors: first, that as the hemophiliac matures, he learns how to take care of himself better, and how to avoid situations that get him into trouble. And secondly, related to the researches reported above, as adolescence passes, the hemophilic boy's psychological conflicts of the kinds mentioned above may lessen: he has a firmer sense of who he is and what he wants to do, a more stable identity.

COUNSELING INTERVENTIONS

In this chapter, we have reviewed some of the psychological and developmental problems of hemophiliacs and their parents.

It is now in order to discuss some counseling methods that can help to overcome or to prevent such problems. In doing so, we do not mean to suggest that every family with a hemophilic member stands in need of intensive professional counseling, or that each growing hemophilic youngster or adult has psychological problems of such magnitude that only "depth" psychotherapy could correct them. Some investigators have indeed emphasized the gravity of the personality difficulties inherent in hemophiliacs and their families. We believe such studies are valuable, but that they have tended to concentrate on extreme cases. The thrust of our own research has been that by-and-large hemophiliacs and their families have done remarkably well, without much professional help or counseling; but that they could do even better and avoid considerable suffering and distress were more help available.

Professional counseling for families may be appropriate from the time the diagnosis of hemophilia is made; or even before maternity, in genetic counseling, where there is a known family history.

The ability of the mother to come to terms with her role as the carrier of the defective gene may require help from the family doctor, a social worker, or other counselor. Marital conflicts, disagreements on methods of bringing up the child, on what to tell relatives and neighbors, on the relationship of the hemophilic child to his siblings—all these are appropriate subjects for counseling, if the parents cannot surmount their psychological difficulties or disagreements themselves. While occasional emotional upsets are to be expected, prolonged and deep ones can result in a strained or abnormal home environment for the growing child, and should be an immediate warning signal for professional help. The latter may be provided by a social worker, psychiatrist, or psychologist at the treatment center; by an outside agency such as a family service agency or mental hygiene clinic, or it may be provided by a hemophilia association or even by other parents.

Group discussion sessions for parents of hemophiliacs can be very valuable, both as a vehicle for necessary information on physical care, on child-rearing practices, and on the psychological needs of hemophiliacs as well as for ventilating the parents' own reactions and problems. Parents learn from one another in such sessions and can often communicate with one another more effectively than with professionals. It is self-evident that those who counsel hemophiliacs need a detailed knowledge of all the physical manifestations, the patterns of psychological development, and the goals of helping the parents to achieve a relaxed and realistic style of behavior toward their son.

The hemophilic youngster's personality develops in response to the limiting effects of his physical disorder, but also, most importantly, in response to the messages he receives from the outside world. In the first instance, these come from his parents, siblings, and other relatives, then from playmates and schoolmates, from teachers, neighbors, and other adults. If these messages are constructive, emphasizing not his disabilities or his differences, but his capacities and his competence, it is not likely that he will stand in need of the same kind of professional help. On the other hand, inconsistent parental handling, prolonging dependency and overprotection, isolation from social experience—all of which are relatively common—can produce severe personality problems which require professional counseling.

For adolescents, who face the problems of identity-establishment, sexual maturation, the choice of a career, and possible separation from parental influences, group and/or individual counseling is frequently desirable. We shall have more to say at a later point about the importance of early and realistic prevocational and vocational counseling.

It is evident, too, that school experience is crucial to the hemophiliac's future. School problems should never be allowed to accumulate, without the parents seeking help from school counselors, psychologists, or other appropriate personnel.

Chapter 5

THE EDUCATION OF HEMOPHILIACS

THE present is a period of great ferment in all levels of education, both in the United States and abroad. Since the first Sputnik—only a decade in the past—major reappraisals of goals, curricula, teaching methods, the respective roles of school, students, parents, and the wider community have gone on ceaselessly. The goals and shape of education are influenced by broad social and technological changes: the knowledge explosion, population pressures, automation, Negro and other minority group strivings, urban deterioration—the catalog is almost endless.

Because of these influences, no one can know with certainty what the future look of education will be in the United States—the only certainty is that there will be changes.

Yet, despite the difficulties of prediction, there are a number of immediate practical problems and special needs in the education of handicapped children in general, hemophiliacs in particular.

These problems have brought increasing emphasis in recent years to the field of special education. This term refers to the giving of instructional service to children who, because of physical, mental, social, or emotional deviation, need some special help in order to operate effectively in the learning situation. Special education in this sense is a recognized specialty in schools of education.

A major principle of special education is that the child's lack or defect should be compensated for by specially devised enrichments to the normal learning situation. These enrichments may take the form of individual or group tutoring, home instruction, or the use of special teaching equipment in classroom, playground, or home. Individualizing the needs of each child while maximizing the development of all the capacities he possesses is basic to special as well as to general education.

The modern concept of learning is that it involves the whole child—senses, muscles, feelings, intellect, observation, and memory. So that if an impairment exists in the organism's apparatus, in any of its modes or pathway to learning, it must be made up for through special effort or attention.

In the case of hemophiliacs there usually are no sense-impairments—as in the case of deaf or blind children—or no intellectual impairments—as in the mentally retarded. Hemophiliacs' deficits and special needs come rather from an accumulated deprivation in ordinary school experience, either through the effects of absence because of hospitalization or disabling illness at home, or because of the school's unwillingness to admit and educate them.

The deprivations that result from frequent and prolonged school absences, or from exclusion, are not solely academic. As the previous chapter has made clear, the isolation of being frequently hospital-bound or home-bound can have damaging effects even on quite young children. Deprivations in social experience, in play, in the stimulation and learning of the skills of social interaction, of getting along with others, of sharing and compromising, of learning the expectations and opportunities in the wider world outside the protected family circle, can all be undesirable by-products of the hemophilic youngster's enforced isolation.

Nursery school, for the hemophilic toddler, is a good idea, for it helps shape the social skills and social competence important at all stages of life. Where possible, hemophilic preschoolers should have the advantages of several hours a day experience in supervised group settings such as day nurseries and kindergartens. Interpretation by physicians can allay the fears of directors and teachers in such settings of any unusual hazards faced in admitting hemophiliacs.

PROBLEMS OF THE SCHOOLS

Public schools' unwillingness to accept hemophiliacs may arise out of fear; some school authorities simply share popular misconceptions about hemophiliacs and exclude them in the belief they will be too great a risk or medical problem. Smaller school districts may have no provisions for home teaching or the newer teaching aids for homebound children, such as closed-circuit television, home and school telephones, and programmed teaching-machines.

Large classes and crowded classrooms are other possible obstacles to the provision of good learning experiences for hemophiliacs. Youngsters having special problems–in the case of hemophiliacs, usually frequent and long absences from school-require more individual attention and encouragement than can be given in a class of thirty-five or forty.

Teacher attitudes may be another problem. The special needs, sensitivities, and possible personality problems of hemophilic youngsters need to be understood to work with them optimally. While some teachers have intuitive understanding of their special needs, or knowledge gained from reading or special education courses, this is by no means universal.

The results of all these interrelated factors have often been reported about hemophiliacs and may be seen in the educational achievement of the 1055 men in our own study.

Let us briefly recapitulate these findings, which were more extensively presented in Chapter 3.

In our study group of 1055, 279 were still in school and 776 were out of school; but complete information was lacking on 123 of the latter.

Of the men out of school, at least 35 percent had not completed high school. Some 24 percent had only a grade school education; while, at the other extreme, 4.25 percent had received a graduate university degree. About 19 percent of the hemophiliacs had had some college training, and about 12 percent were college graduates.

The figures in Table IX compare hemophiliacs with the general male population in the United States.

The median number of school years completed for United States males in 1965 was 11.7 years; for our study group, it was 10.9.

While, of itself, this difference is not too significant, it should be borne in mind that the average United States figures above are reduced by the lower educational status of Negroes, which in 1965 averaged about half that of white American males. Taking this into account, the school achievement of hemophiliacs does come out significantly lower than the general United States average.

TABLE IX

Years of School Completed	*General Population**	*653 Hemophiliacs*
Elementary school		
less than 7	18.8	7.09
7 – 9	15.9	15.46
High school		
10 – 11	17.3	11.73
12 years (or graduated)	27.1	26.55
College		
1 – 3 years	9.3	7.47
4 years or more	12.7	11.74

*Source: *Statistical Abstract of the United States,* 155. 1966, p. 113.

From extensive discussions with hemophilic students and their families as well as with teachers and school administrators, Dr. Frances O'Connor, an authority on special education, has summarized some broad conclusions on the education of hemophiliacs as follows:

1. In general, with a few exceptions, children with hemophilia are achieving below the chronological age expectation and below their actual intellectual ability level.
2. Children with hemophilia appear to experience school careers marked by attendance gaps and inconsistencies in programming. Some youngsters, particularly the intellectually gifted, can compensate through independent study if assisted by family guidance.
3. Teachers in both regular grades and special education programs are not adequately prepared to cope with or even accept comfortably the youngster with hemophilia.
4. Some school administrators hesitate to accommodate hemophiliacs in their total school programs, owing to undue fear and consequent "overprotection," resulting in forced nonparticipation of the child.
5. Comprehensive and coordinated school programs for hemophilic children requiring instruction in either or both hospitals or their own homes are relatively rare.
6. Parents, in general, want their sons to attend school in the regular classroom rather than to have them singled out for special classes or special programs. Parental attitudes, which vary from family to

family, influence school success.

7. Developmental and/or remedial academic programs offered to hemophiliacs on a tutorial basis, as an extra part of the total educational provision, would be helpful in compensating for school absences.

8. Serious question is raised relative to the quality of school and vocational guidance given to teen-agers with hemophilia(4).

Dr. O'Connor's analysis raises sharply the issue of the general approach and the special provisions needed to upgrade the quality of education received by hemophiliacs.

Since education is viewed as a local responsibility in the United States, improvements will be brought about primarily at the initiative of local school boards. Through recent legislation, the United States Office of Education has established a division to encourage special education, by grants for teacher training and research in the development of new teaching aids and devices. But utilizing these resources depends on the motivation of local school systems to improve their special education programs. This is a many-sided task; it can be aided by the work of parents and local hemophilia associations, by physicians, social workers and counselors familiar with the problems, and by well-timed interpretive publicity.

As a minimum it would seem that local school boards should do the following things:

1. In collaboration with universities, develop standards and teacher training programs for special education, which will insure that teachers of handicapped children will have understanding of their special needs, problems, and conditions of learning.

2. Acquire realistic knowledge of hemophiliacs as being fully educable in the standard school setting, although presenting needs for some restricted physical activity.

3. In collaboration with hospitals, work out instructional programs for children who have lengthy periods of hospitalization.

4. Develop instruction methods for children who must be homebound for more than one week at a time, through use of home teachers, closed-circuit TV, home-school telephones, programmed teaching machines.

5. In the absence of the above, arrange for individual and group remedial and tutoring of children who have missed substantial

school time.

6. In conjunction with state vocational-rehabilitation departments, arrange for early prevocational testing and counseling of hemophilic students. Ideally, this would be available from junior-high age on, since early choice and preparation for a career can be important for the physically handicapped. Rehabilitation services that provide counseling, training, and placement should be available to all teen-agers who wish to use them, and should be coordinated with academic programs.

Underlying these recommendations are the concepts of the unity and continuity of educational processes. For any child, handicapped or not, education is a development of the personality and the skills of social living, in addition to cognitive or academic learning. Such learning should start with the group experiences of preschool education, progress through the elementary and secondary levels, so that the growing child is equipped with the necessary knowledge and tools to make a realistic choice for his adult career, and to pursue the necessary further training. Ideally, this would call for close cooperation between the health care, social service, educational and vocational agencies and professionals, as well as consultation with the hemophiliac's family, and his own desires.

THE QUESTION OF SPECIAL SCHOOLS

In the light of all the problems and deficiencies in present educational facilities—far short of the ideal situation sketched above—it is not surprising that in some countries, hemophilia associations, parent groups, and physicians have organized special boarding schools for hemophiliacs. Advocates of such schools believe that through them the educational problems of hemophiliacs can be most efficiently overcome, with the least expenditure of effort.

A principle underlying the creation of special boarding schools for severely affected hemophilic boys is that the school can be run in close association with an advanced hemophilia treatment center. The first known boarding school especially designed for hemophilic boys was opened by the French Red Cross in 1958, taking boys from six to fifteen years of age. Subsequently two more schools were opened in France, one near Paris and one in the Savoy region. These schools are reported to be a great success—even though boarding schools are not a tradition in France—and there are long waiting lists for admission. Parents are reported to believe that the accessibility of facilities to the schools has resulted in early treatment and prevention of hemarthroses.

England, which has experienced some of the same difficulties in adequate education for hemophiliacs as the United States, has one boarding school which admits severe hemophiliacs, and a group of Oxford physicians and parents are attempting to establish another one.

As far as is known, there is no strong movement in this direction in the United States or Canada, but there is interest in studying the European experience. The general pros and cons are clear: the complete integration of handicapped and nonhandicapped youngsters is the ideal of our educational efforts; segregation is seen as having negative psychological aspects; but on the other hand, more continuous education, closely linked to preventive medical care, can be given in this way.

In a complex situation, there are few absolutes, and compromise is a part of all living. As education is so crucial a factor in adjustment, its potential for hemophiliacs should be maximized. Local action, adapted to local circumstances, would seem to be the key to progress.

Chapter 6

MAKING A LIVING

SATISFYING work experience has long been considered a cornerstone and major ingredient of a successful life. Freud spoke of "the ability to work" and " the ability to love" as two chief signs of a healthy personality, and most psychologists, most theologians, and indeed most laymen would agree.

In recent years, the rehabilitation movement has drawn considerable attention to the work problems of physically disabled people. Much public education, professional effort, and research have been devoted to the ideas that the physically disabled can and should work; that they often need, however, some special training and some modifications of the work environment to bring this about. Employers, schools, unions, families, and, ultimately, disabled people themselves have been the targets of the efforts to promote and popularize these ideas.

Hemophiliacs have the same needs as other people for work satisfactions and the material and psychological benefits that come from it. But frequently they require some special help in the choice of a suitable profession or occupation; training for the skills needed in it; interpretation to employers, toward a safe working environment, and in provisions for rehabilitation and placement.

Until 1963-64, the work situation of hemophiliacs had not been studied in depth. At that time, the writer conducted the already-cited study of the social and vocational situation of adult hemophiliacs, through a project financed by the U.S. Vocational Rehabilitation Administration.

Findings of our pioneering study of the work situation of hemophiliacs will be presented rather extensively in this and the next chapter, since they represent the most complete information presently available on the subject. More recent studies will also be alluded to.

EMPLOYMENT STATUS

In general the hemophiliacs in our study showed a higher number and proportion who were employed, with a more normal vocational history than had been anticipated. In fact, most of the men in the study were either working or were still in school. Only sixty participants (about 8 percent of those who had left school) were classified as "Never Employed"; most of these were in the youngest age group, between sixteen and nineteen years, or the early twenties. In view of this age distribution, it seemed likely that some of the never employed would be employed at some time in the future.

The subjects in the study were classified into four main groups with regard to employment status: *(1) the employed, (2) the unemployed, (3) the never-employed* and *(4) those still in school* (some of whom had returned to school after a period of working). The self-employed constituted a subgroup within the employed and unemployed groups. These four groups will be considered separately in Table X.

TABLE X

EMPLOYMENT STATUS, 1,055 HEMOPHILIACS

Status	*Number*	*Percent*
Currently employed	552	52
Currently unemployed	152	14
Retired	12	1
Still in school	279	29
Never employed	60	6
	1,055	99

The currently employed, the still in school, and the retired, comprising 82 percent of the subjects, can be characterized as living in a "normal" manner with regard to their vocational status. Further, 23 percent of the currently unemployed had held their most recent position for from four to twenty years, so that some of them may be considered as temporarily unemployed or as approaching retirement. Thus, the study indicates that *it is not only possible, but also not unusual for hemophiliacs to be engaged full-time in gainful employment* despite the handicaps of their physical condition and the consequent deficits of education and training.

The unemployment rate for the men in the study (20% of the 776 who were not still in school) was far higher, however, than the 4.6 percent reported for their age group in the 1960 Census report(19).

A significantly greater proportion (22%) of the unemployed compared to the employed (6%) had held *part-time* jobs as their last employment. Of the employed, 22 percent were self-employed; while 11 percent of the unemployed were self-employed in their last position.

Of those still in school, most were in the younger ages—93 percent in the teens and twenties. About 50 percent were currently working while attending school, or had worked at some time on full-time, part-time, or vacation and summer jobs.

TABLE XI

NUMBER OF MONTHS EMPLOYED
IN PRESENT OR MOST RECENT POSITION

	Employed (N = 564)*		*Unemployed (N = 152)*	
	Number	*Percent*	*Number*	*Percent*
3 months or less	33	6	33	22
4 – 11 months	63	11	36	24
12 months – 2 years	96	17	25	16
25 months – 4 years	73	13	11	7
49 months – 7 years	80	14	9	6
85 months – 10 years	61	11	9	6
121 months – 15 years	50	9	13	9
over 15 years	78	14	4	3
No information	30	5	12	8
	564	100	152	100

*Includes retired (N = 12)

Another surprising finding was that of those who were not still in school (N=776) 10 percent had served in the armed forces. Several respondents stated the Service had taken them not believing they were hemophiliacs, or because the Service doctors were unfamiliar with the disease. Some had been allowed to enlist voluntarily.

The majority of the employed hemophiliacs showed a high degree of job stability in that many had remained on one job for a long period of time as illustrated in Table XI. The currently employed differed markedly from the unemployed, with the latter group far less stable in terms of remaining on the job.

OCCUPATIONS

The occupations reported by the hemophiliacs in the study are listed in Table XII and show a very wide range. The more inclusive categories in this table, such as white collar, technical, clerical, services, and workers include positions that differ in degrees of skill, education required, amount of responsibility, and physical activity.

TABLE XII

OCCUPATIONAL DISTRIBUTION OF RESPONDENTS

Occupations	*Employed-Retired (N = 564)*		*Unemployed (N = 152)*	
	Number	*Percent*	*Number*	*Percent*
Professional	59	10	3	2
Executive or owners, large business	32	6	0	0
Manager or owner, small business	41	7	6	4
Arts	18	3	2	1
Supervisors	16	3	5	3
White collar	93	16	18	12
Technical, craftsmen	71	13	15	10
Clerical	70	12	22	14
Services	38	7	26	17
Laborers (Skilled, semi-, unskilled)	100	18	40	26
Other	6	1	3	2
No information	20	4	12	8
	564	100	152	99

The technical category implies a requirement for a specific kind of technical skill or knowledge, unlike other categories such as clerical, which refers to paper-and-pencil work, or some kind of record-keeping function. The technical category contains diversified kinds of occupations which may have little relation to one another beyond the idea that they require some kind and degree of specific skill.

Occupational *differences* between the employed and the unemployed are also shown in Table XII. Some comparisons with the occupational distribution in the general population males, aged fourteen years and over, are of interest. The 1960 Census shows the following percentages in the general population: professional-technical (our professional), 4 percent; clerical, 5 percent; laborers, 19 percent; craftsmen (our technical, craftsmen), 10 percent; The employed hemophiliacs in the study showed a higher percentage than the national average in these categories except laborers, where they were about equal.

Perhaps the most important and surprising finding from our study is that hemophiliacs are by no means confined to sedentary occupations, nor to tasks which require little or no training. Many of the laborers, and among them individuals with severe hemophilic involvement, were working at such physically active occupations as longshoring, road maintenance, housepainting and welding. Among the service personnel were waiters, delivery and errand boys, and gas station attendants. It is likely that such occupations tend to increase the frequency of hemorrhages, either by actual injury such as a blow or a cut, or by stresses on areas of the body, which might lead to spontaneous internal bleeding. A common finding is that occupations which require the individual to be on his feet a great deal, either standing or walking, lead to severe joint involvements. Overuse of particular body parts even in such seemingly sedentary work as watch repair can lead to joint hemorrhages; several watch repairmen who answered the study questionnaire complained of hemophilic arthropathies in the finger joints, necessitating abandoning that trade. Despite the apparent relationship between certain stressful kinds of physical activity and vulnerability to hemorrhaging, no real relationship was found between the severity of illness (measured in the study by number of hemorrhages per year) and the kind of occupation. This fact suggests two conclusions: (1) while bodily stress may influence the particular site where hemorrhaging occurs, it does not necessarily affect its overall incidence and (2) severity of illness (except at the extreme) does not appreciably influence the choice of occupation.

INCOME

Table XIII presents the weekly income level for the employed-unemployed in their present or most recent job (these data were gathered from June 1963 to July 1964).

TABLE XIII

INCOME OF HEMOPHILIACS

Income	*Employed* (N = 564)*		*Unemployed (N = 152)*	
	Number	*Percent*	*Number*	*Percent*
Under $50 per week	74	13	64	42
$50 to $75 per week	110	20	37	24
$76 to $100 per week	115	20	24	16
Over $100	227	40	16	11
No information	38	7	11	7
	564	100	152	100

*Includes retired (N = 12)

The distribution is fairly even for the four income levels for the employed. The large number of above $100 weekly income results from the low ceiling, reflecting the researchers' expectations prior to the study. It had been assumed that the income level of hemophiliacs would not be parallel to that of the nonhemophilic population, but would be significantly lower. Incomes of the employed hemophiliacs, however, tended to be higher than those for males fourteen years of age and over in the general population. The most nearly comparable table from the 1960 Census showed the following: income $1-$2,499–30 percent; $2,500-$3,999–15 percent; $4,000-$4999–13 percent; $5,000 and over–42 percent(19). The unemployed in our study showed a far lower income level in their last employment than the employed.

Thus, the majority of hemophiliacs in the study can and do successfully fulfill their roles as family breadwinners. Married hemophiliacs tend to take their place as the head of the household and are not usually dependent on their wives to support them, although the wives may be employed to the same extent as are wives of nonhemophiliacs.

UNEMPLOYMENT, AND COMPARISONS BETWEEN THE EMPLOYED AND THE UNEMPLOYED

While we found that 82 percent of the total sample were employed, retired, or still in school, the study also showed that of those eligible for employment (not still in school) about 27 percent were unemployed or had never been employed. It has already been pointed out that some hemophiliacs had been unemployed for only a short period of time and therefore in the long run might have a relatively "normal" vocational picture, and that a large percentage of the never employed were in their teens and early twenties.

Nevertheless, there appear to be a sizable number of the unemployed and never-employed who, when the above factors of age and length of unemployment are considered, can be described as chronically unemployed. It seems valuable, therefore, to present the descriptive data regarding unemployment and go on to discuss the differences between the chronically unemployed and the employed with regard to such factors as severity of illness, educational achievement, and employment history.

Frequency Of Unemployment

The respondents were asked to state the number of times they had been unemployed since leaving school, the length of each period of unemployment and the reasons, as indicated in Table XIV.

According to Table XIV very few of the employed had had frequent unemployment; whereas this was less true for the unemployed.

TABLE XIV

NUMBER OF TIMES UNEMPLOYED

Number of Times Unemployed	*Employed/Retired (N = 564)*		*Unemployed (N = 152)*	
	Number	*Percent*	*Number*	*Percent*
No unemployment reported	356	63	54	36
One time	79	14	15	10
Two times	36	6	14	9
Three times	16	3	15	10
Four to eight times	28	5	13	9
"Several"	17	3	17	11
Indicated periods of unemployment, but not number of times	32	6	24	16
	564	100	152	101

Duration of Unemployment

Table XV shows the duration of unemployment for one of the periods of unemployment listed by those who responded to the question. As would be expected, the unemployed indicated long periods more frequently than the employed.

TABLE XV

LENGTH OF UNEMPLOYMENT FOR FIRST PERIOD LISTED

Number of Months	*Employed/Retired (N = 208)**		*Unemployed (N = 98)**	
	Number	*Percent*	*Number*	*Percent*
1 month	18	9	3	3
2 months	25	12	7	7
3 – 4 months	45	22	11	11
5 – 8 months	42	20	14	14
9 – 16 months	22	11	11	11
17 – 32 months	9	4	9	9
33 months to over 65 months	14	7	18	18
Indicated periods of unemployment, but not number of months	33	16	25	26
	208	101	98	99

*Number reporting periods of unemployment

While Table XV is clearly incomplete in the amount of information it provides regarding duration of unemployment, by utilizing dates given for last job for most of the unemployed, we were able to determine the length of time since their most recent employment, as shown in Table XVI.

TABLE XVI

LENGTH OF TIME
SINCE MOST RECENT EMPLOYMENT FOR THE UNEMPLOYED (N = 152)

Length of Time	*Number*	*Percent*
Under 3 months	26	17
3 to under 7 months	25	16
7 months to 1 year	26	17
13 months to 2 years	16	11
25 months to 3 years	8	5
37 months to under 7 years	19	13
7 years and over	22	14
No information	10	7
	152	100

Table XVI shows that about 43 percent of the unemployed had not worked for at least a year, and about 32 percent had not worked for at least two years.

Reasons for Unemployment

Table XVII shows the reasons for their last unemployment, as listed by the respondents.

TABLE XVII

REASONS FOR LAST UNEMPLOYMENT

Reasons	*Employed/Retired (N = 208)*		*Unemployed (N = 98)*	
	Number	*Percent*	*Number*	*Percent*
Health—hemophilia	62	30	41	41
Health—not hemophilia	12	6	5	5
Accident (whether or not hemophilia complicated)	6	3	2	2
Looking for better job	23	11	3	3
Job not available	56	27	18	18
No one would hire because of hemophilia	4	2	3	3
Reason not known	43	21	26	26
	206	100	98	98

For both groups, hemophilia was seen as a major reason for unemployment; however for the employed it was not the most frequent reason; rather they stated that most frequently jobs were not available. The unemployed gave hemophilia-related reasons for their unemployment to a considerably greater extent than did the employed. This suggests that the unemployed are or feel more handicapped by their hemophilia than the employed.

Reasons for Leaving Jobs

Table XVIII provides information regarding job termination for the respondents' most recent position.

In general, the most frequent reasons for leaving jobs were health, employer cutbacks, and the respondent's finding a better job. Table XVIII, however, reveals some significant differences between the employed and the unemployed. The employed most frequently left jobs because they had found a better one; the unemployed most frequently for health reasons—41 percent had left their last job because of health. The unemployed also had a higher percentage of temporary positions and were fired more often for hemophilia-related reasons.

THE CHRONICALLY UNEMPLOYED: SUCCESSFUL VERSUS UNSUCCESSFUL

Defining the Groups

So far we have discussed some differences in the job experiences of employed and unemployed hemophiliacs. Other differences between the two groups may also be examined, particularly those that affect "success" for purposes of comparison. Our study used the idea of "success" in these comparisons, the single criterion being whether or not the person was employed at the time of data-gathering. If currently employed, the subject was considered "successful."

Unemployment of seven months and over was designated as lengthy and classed the hemophiliac in the "unsuccessful" group. Comparisons were then made between (1) *successful:* employed,

TABLE XVIII

REASONS FOR RESIGNATION AND DISCHARGE FROM JOBS

Reasons	*Previous Position*		*Most Recent Position*
	*Employed** *(N = 440)*	*Unemployed* *(N = 119)*	*Unemployed* *(N = 167)***
	%	%	%
Resigned			
Found a better job	31	11	1
Wanted to look for a better job	5	4	4
To return to school	3	3	2
Job ended, temporary	6	10	8
Health reasons	12	23	41
Work dangerous for hemophilia	2	6	2
Not enough pay	6	2	4
Changed residence	2	3	2
Poor relationship with			2
boss	3	3	
Other	3	4	2
To go into business for			0
self	2	0	0
	75	69	68
Discharged			
Cut back, or employer went out of business	16	18	15
Employee's work production low	1	0	2
Employer thought respondent needed more training	<1	2	1
Employer thought working conditions bad for hemophiliac	1	2	4
Employer found out about respondent's hemophilia, absences due to hemophilia, other hemophilia causes	3	9	9
	22	31	31

*Includes retired (N = 12).

**N's are number of responses counted, since some respondents gave more than one answer. Respondents who gave no answer are not included.

twenty-five years of age and over. (There were 447 of these.) and (2) *unsuccessful:* unemployed and never-employed, twenty-five years of age and over, unemployed at least seven months (105 individuals).

The "unsuccessful" in the study comprised about 19 percent of the potential working group, twenty-five years of age and over.

Eighty-four unemployed and twenty-one never-employed were in the unsuccessful group. Retired workers (N=12) were included with the employed since their vocational adjustment can be considered similar to that of the latter, retirement being a normal vocational pattern.

Severity of Illness in Relation to Success

On every measure of severity of illness, the unsuccessful were found to have a significantly greater proportion of persons of high severity than the successful. According to the Index of Severity used in the study, less than 25 percent of the unsuccessful, but almost 50 percent of the successful are of low severity. About 30 percent of the unsuccessful and 16 percent of the successful are of high severity. The remainder in both groups were of intermediate severity.

About 23 percent of the entire sample reported no arthropathies. However, only 3 percent of the unsuccessful reported no arthropathies; 82 percent had them in two or more sites. Among the successful, 20 percent had no arthropathies, 56 percent had arthropathies in two or more sites.

Approximately 42 percent of the unsuccessful as compared with 22 percent of the successful had used a wheelchair at some time in their lives.

The respondents were asked to state how they would rate their health other than with respect to hemophilia. About 56 percent of the successful rated their health as "very good," 33 percent as "good," and 11 percent as "fair-poor." Only 33 percent of the unsuccessful rated their health as "very good," 22 percent as "good," and 44 percent as "fair-poor."

About 44 percent of the unsuccessful listed specific medical problems other than hemophilia and about 33 percent of the successful did so. The unsuccessful reported a greater number of hospitalizations during the past two years.

Employment and Income of the Successful and the Unsuccessful

A total of 74 percent of the unsuccessful stated that they could not work full-time; although, of those who held a previous position and who responded to the question, 64 percent had held full-time positions. Of the successful, 17 percent said they could not work full-time, but 95 percent in fact held full-time jobs.

The unsuccessful tended to have held their last position for a shorter time than the successful had held their present one; 30 percent of the unsuccessful had worked on that job for seven years or longer, compared with 44 percent of the successful. Of the unsuccessful, 24 percent had worked for eleven months or less, compared to 11 percent for the successful.

Differences in income between the groups were great, as indicated in Table XIX.

TABLE XIX

INCOME ON PRESENT JOB FOR SUCCESSFUL, MOST RECENT JOB FOR UNSUCCESSFUL

	Successful (N = 447)		*Unsuccessful (N = 105)*	
	Number	*Percent*	*Number*	*Percent*
Under $50.00 per week	45	10	37	35
$50 – $75 per week	63	14	15	14
$76 – $100 per week	91	20	13	12
Over $100 per week	215	48	8	8
No information (includes the never-employed for the unsuccessful)	33	7	32	30
	447	99	105	99

Table XIX demonstrates the circularity of problems faced by many hemophiliacs. Hemophilia is an expensive disease; and the more severe the case, the more expensive it is. Also, the more severe the case, the less likely it is that the subject can work and earn regularly.

Table XX shows incomes for the low and high-severe groups.

TABLE XX

INCOME ON PRESENT OR
MOST RECENT JOB FOR LOW AND HIGH-SEVERE RESPONDENTS

	Low-Severe (N = 310)		*High-Severe (N = 159)*	
	Number	*Percent*	*Number*	*Percent*
Under $50.00 per week	36	12	46	29
$50 – $75 per week	60	19	36	23
$76 – $100 per week	59	19	22	14
Over $100 per week	121	42	25	16
No information or never employed	24	8	30	19
	310	100	159	101

These findings demonstrate a pattern, one which begins early in life, at the time the hemophiliac is of school age and preparing for his vocational future and continuing to the time he is of working age. Reflected in this pattern is the effectiveness of the hemophiliac's job performance, his ability to be physically present on the job, and his earning capacity. It is clear, of course, that not all hemophiliacs who are "severe" cases have low incomes or are otherwise vocationally unsuccessful–wide individual differences appear in vocational adjustment to the degree of severity.

Great differences were found between the successful and the unsuccessful in types of occupation. Virtually no professionals and executives were found among the latter group; while about 20 percent of the successful were in these occupations. Table XXI provides further occupational comparisons and indicates that the unsuccessful had held jobs requiring less education or training than the successful.

TABLE XXI

OCCUPATIONS OF
SUCCESSFUL AND UNSUCCESSFUL RESPONDENTS

Occupation	*Successful (N = 435)**		*Unsuccessful (N = 77)**	
	Number	*Percent*	*Number*	*Percent*
Professional	54	12	1	1
Executive	32	7	0	0
Manager-owner, small business	36	8	5	6
Arts	15	3	1	1
Supervisors	15	3	4	5
White collar, level I	62	14	7	9
White collar, level II	15	3	3	4
Clerical, level I	18	4	1	1
Clerical, level II	33	8	10	13
Technical, level I	28	6	6	8
Technical, level II	25	6	3	4
Services	12	3	8	10
Drivers	15	3	9	12
Skilled-semiskilled worker	50	11	8	10
Unskilled worker	21	5	9	12
Other	4	1	2	3
	435	97**	77	99

*Number in each group for whom occupational information was available.
**Rounding errors.

Differences in Education and Training

Amount of education is another significant difference between successful and unsuccessful hemophiliacs. A cross-tabulation of the highest grade achieved by the successful and unsuccessful is revealed in Table XXII.

At least 52 percent of the unsuccessful did not complete high school, and this percentage would probably be higher if there were data for those who gave no information.

The groups also differed markedly in their reasons for discontinuing their education. The unsuccessful quit school because of health reasons (44%), because they completed their course (22%), and because, they had been held back in school or saw no sense in continuing, because of health (17%). The successful quit school because they completed their course (38%)

and for financial reasons (21%). Only 16 percent of the successful left school because of health reasons and 12 percent because they were held back or discouraged. Only 10 percent of the unsuccessful quit school for financial reasons.

About 12 percent of both groups said they had received help from the Vocational Rehabilitation Service. Three fourths of the unsuccessful had received financial aid from some source; while only 42 percent of the successful had received such help.

TABLE XXII

HIGHEST GRADE ACHIEVED BY
THE SUCCESSFUL AND UNSUCCESSFUL RESPONDENTS

Highest Grade	*Successful (N = 447)*		*Unsuccessful (N = 105)*	
	Number	*Percent*	*Number*	*Percent*
6th grade and under	21	5	19	18
7th to 9th grades	68	15	25	24
10th and 11th grades	50	11	11	10
12th grade or graduated from high school	118	26	21	20
Some college or university	59	13	5	5
Graduated from college or university	34	8	1	1
Graduate school, or completed advanced degree	42	9	1	1
No information	55	12	22	21
	447	99	105	100

Differences in Personal and Social Characteristics of the Successful and Unsuccessful

The differences between the two groups were also pursued into other areas, with interesting results.

1. Marital Status, Living Conditions

Of the successful, 77 percent were married, 2 percent were divorced or separated, 1 percent were widowed, and 19 percent were single. This distribution is in contrast to the unsuccessful, of whom 44 percent were married, 9 percent divorced or separated, and 48 percent single. Forty-three (43%) of the unsuccessful lived with their parents, 6 percent lived with other relatives, and 7 percent lived alone. Of the successful, 13 percent lived with parents, 3 percent with other relatives, and 6 percent lived alone. The successful who were or had been married were far more likely to have had children than were the married unsuccessful.

2. Leisure-time Activities

Most of the hemophiliacs stated they had hobbies; however, the unsuccessful reported fewer interests and hobbies than did the successful.

The successful listed more leisure-time activities than did the unsuccessful; many more of the latter listed no leisure-time activities at all. The activity level of the successful seemed to be higher than that of the unsuccessful; the unsuccessful showed a greater tendency toward solitary and passive activities.

These findings regarding personal and social characteristics of the successful and unsuccessful indicate real differences between the groups in their modes of life, not merely occupational differences. The unemployed or unsuccessful give the impression of a greater passivity and a more resigned or negative outlook.

Differences Among the Success-Severity Groups

Because the degree to which severity had bearing on the above-described differences between successful and unsuccessful was unknown, four success-severity groups were formed for comparison. That is, the two success groups were divided into four as follows:

1. Successful low-severe (N=210).
2. Successful high-severe (N=70).
3. Unsuccessful low-severe (N=26).
4. Unsuccessful high-severe (N=31).

These groups were formed by combining the variables of success-nonsuccess with the Index of Severity. Thus, for example, the successful low-severe were employed, twenty-five years of age and over who rated low on the Index of Severity. The unsuccessful high-severe were unemployed–never-employed, twenty-five years of age and over, who had been unemployed for at least seven months and who rated high on the Index of Severity.

We found on other measures of severity, e.g. occurrence of arthropathies and number and duration of hemorrhages before age sixteen, that the unsuccessful low showed a higher severity than do the successful low and that the unsuccessful high-severe measure higher on the other severity measures than do the successful high. This finding is, in itself, of importance in that it indicates that one of the most consistent factors related to success-nonsuccess is reported state of health.

Nevertheless, there were seventy respondents who were high severe and who were successful, and it is important to compare that group and the unsuccessful of low and of high severity. What are some of the differences between them and the unsuccessful in attitudes, work experiences, education, and other social experiences? In general, the successful highs measured higher on the severity measures than did the unsuccessful lows, yet they have been able to function adequately according to the criteria of this study. We found, for example, that 87 percent of the successful highs had two or more arthropathies, only 1 percent reporting "none." A total of 98 percent of the unsuccessful high and 80 percent of the unsuccessful low had two or more arthropathies. The successful low had 43 percent in that category. The successful high, then, rate very high on number of hemorrhages per year reported and on occurrence and number of arthropathies.

Personal and Social Characteristics of the Success-Severity Groups

Different patterns of living separate the four success-severity groups, so that it might be said that a characteristic picture emerges once the individual is placed within one of the groups. On the one hand, the hemophiliac may be of high or low severity, but is employed, physically and socially active, married, has children, and in general has a relatively cheerful and constructive outlook. On the other hand there are hemophiliacs of comparably low severity, who have consistent patterns of unemployment, who are inactive and socially withdrawn, likely to be unmarried, who are undereducated, and who indicate gloomy and pessimistic views of life in their verbal reports.

Tables XXIII and XXIV reflect some of these differences. It can be seen that while the successful lows have the greatest tendency to be married, the successful highs also have a high proportion who are married. The unsuccessful lows, if married, have the least tendency to have children, while the unsuccessful highs are about the same as the successful groups in that respect. Both unsuccessful groups are less likely to marry than are the successful.

TABLE XXIII

MARITAL STATUS OF SUCCESS-SEVERITY GROUPS

Success-Severity	*Marital Status*			
	Single %	*Married* %	*Divorced-Separated* %	*Widowed* %
Successful low (N = 210)	16	81	1	1
Successful high (N = 70)	27	71	1	0
Unsuccessful low (N = 26)	31	61	8	0
Unsuccessful high (N = 31)	51	42	6	0

Among the unsuccessful lows, 46 percent discontinued their education because of health, and 17 percent because they had completed their studies. The successful highs had 27 percent who left school because of health, and 39 percent because of course completion. The unsuccessful highs show the highest percentage who quit school for hemophilia reasons, about 80 percent.

Despite the relatively lower severity of the unsuccessful lows, these findings illustrate that this group appears early in life to have developed a pattern of considering themselves more handicapped by their hemophilia than have the successful highs.

The unsuccessful lows have only 29 percent who rate their health (other than respect to hemophilia) as "very good" and 33 percent who rate it as "fair-poor." The successful high, on the other hand, have 63 percent who rate their health as "very good" and only 7 percent as "fair-poor." This item was entirely subjective, and may or may not reflect the individuals' actual state of health, other than hemophilia. It is interesting that the successful highs had the highest percentage of all four groups who rated their health as "very good" and that 54 percent of the unsuccessful lows did not list any other specific health complaint, although only 29 percent said their health was "very good."

From these findings we might hypothesize that among hemophiliacs there is a small group of men who, since school age or before, have emphasized to themselves the disabling nature of their illness and who have dropped out of the mainstream of living. Such attitudes should be apparent and detectable by school authorities, vocational rehabilitation counselors, and medical personnel. Dropping out of school, especially for those whose illness is objectively not disabling, can be most destructive, since later adjustment is highly related to school achievement.

There is another group who, despite a higher incidence of more severe physical involvement, tend to de-emphasize their physical condition–almost to deny it–and who are more goal-oriented. This is the successful high-severe group.

Large differences were also found between the unsuccessful lows and the other groups with regard to leisure-time activities. The unsuccessful lows listed fewer activities (35 percent listed no activities, compared to 10 percent for unsuccessful highs) and had the highest percentage listing sedentary activities and the highest tendency to solitary activities.

The successful highs were somewhat more inactive than the successful lows, but far more active than both of the unsuccessful groups.

Employment Characteristics of the Success-Severity Groups

Of the twenty-six persons in the group of unsuccessful lows, four had never been employed, and six of the thirty-one in the unsuccessful highs had never been employed.

Most of the unsuccessful feel they cannot work full-time; 90 percent of the unsuccessful highs and 68 percent of the unsuccessful lows say they cannot, compared to 28 percent for the successful highs. The unsuccessful, particularly the high severity group, had larger percentages who worked part-time on their most recent job than did the successful groups.

Predictably, the unsuccessful group as a whole had lower incomes than did the successful groups, with the unsuccessful highs most extreme in this respect.

Table XXIV shows the percentages for the four success-severity groups in the most frequently listed occupational categories.

TABLE XXIV

OCCUPATIONS OF THE SUCCESS-SEVERITY GROUPS

Occupation	*Success-Severity*			
	*Succ-Low (N = 204)** %	*Succ-High (N = 69)* %	*Unsucc-Low (N = 21)* %	*Unsucc-High (N = 23)* %
Professional	12	13	0	0
Executive	7	6	0	0
Mgr.-owner business	8	13	10	9
White collar, I	13	13	5	4
White collar, II	4	1	0	4
Technical, I	7	4	5	9
Technical, II	5	4	5	4
Clerical, I	3	7	0	0
Clerical, II	5	13	14	13
Services	3	0	10	13
Drivers	4	1	19	13
Skilled-semiskilled labor	12	9	0	13
Unskilled labor	6	7	24	4

*N's are numbers of respondents who answered the question. Some occupations are not not listed, e.g. artists, supervisors, "other."

Table XXIV demonstrates that, in terms of a rough indexing, the unsuccessful lows have a lower occupational level than do the other three groups. They tend to have high percentages in the services, drivers, unskilled labor, and in the lower clerical category. The successful highs do not differ greatly from the successful lows, except that they have a greater proportion of clerical workers. The unsuccessful highs differ from the unsuccessful lows in that the former have more skilled and semiskilled workers and fewer unskilled workers.

The unsuccessful lows, then, appear to be the least successful in terms of occupational level, although they tended to have higher incomes than did the unsuccessful highs. This is probably because the unsuccessful highs had a larger proportion working part-time on their most recent jobs.

Chapter 7

SOME SPECIAL CONDITIONS: HEMOPHILIA AND WORK

THE previous chapter has described some of the conditions and problems faced by the hemophiliac in his work status. Considering the extent of their problems, a surprisingly high proportion of hemophiliacs function effectively in the labor market, despite disabilities from the illness, low educational achievement, and the added burden of discrimination by employers. Relatively little help in finding jobs from governmental agencies was reported in our study; rather hemophiliacs tend to obtain their jobs in the same manner as the unhandicapped—through the undefined method of "job hunting."

FINDING JOBS

The two principal ways in which the respondents found their jobs were by such "job hunting" or through family and friends. A small percentage (5%) found them through public agencies and 5 percent through their schools.

About 12 percent of the respondents had had some contact with their state vocational rehabilitation service, receiving vocational counseling, training and/or aid in furthering their education. Thus, the vast majority of the hemophiliacs had received no vocational counseling or special vocational training.

The most frequent kind of occupational training received was watch repairing, which some hemophiliacs found unsatisfactory in that the income tended to be low and overuse of the fingers sometimes resulted in arthritic-like conditions of the finger joints.

DISCLOSURE TO EMPLOYER AND EMPLOYER ATTITUDES

In addition to inadequate preparation and difficulties in finding and keeping jobs, the major problem faced by many hemophiliacs is employer attitudes. While some hemophiliacs have found employers who are sympathetic to their problems, and a small number (3%) work for their families, the great majority have had bitter and frustrating experiences in job hunting.

Most hemophiliacs confront the dilemma of either informing the employer of their condition and risking the possibility of being refused the job, or of withholding information and jeopardizing their status because of subsequent illness. Some hemophiliacs have an aversion to withholding the truth from employers, with the result that they have frequently been turned down for jobs. Others disclose because, having tried both methods, they feel disclosure is preferable, since they are apt to lose the job later on because of unexplained absenteeism.

According to our findings, about 31 percent do not tell employers; 69 percent of the respondents did disclose their hemophilia.

Of 128 unemployed who responded to the question, 64 percent said they had told their most recent employers of their hemophilia, while 71 percent of the 462 employed responding had done so. The greater tendency for the unemployed to withhold information could result in a greater tendency to be discharged from their positions once the employer learned of their condition, or because of inexplicably poor performance or absence from the job.

It appears that most hemophiliacs begin their working careers by telling employers of their condition, some later deciding not to do so because of the frequency with which they have been turned down for jobs. The unemployed state they have had far more experiences of this kind than have the employed. Of the employed, 51 percent state they never tell employers that they have hemophilia. Of the unemployed, only 27 percent say they have never been turned down for that reason, while 24 percent say they have never told employers. In addition, of the unemployed who have been refused jobs, most have been refused very frequently.

The hemophiliac who dissembles in this way, according to the self-reports, frequently feels anxiety and guilt. If he has arthropathies, he is forced to manufacture plausible excuses for such obvious handicaps. Some say that they have had polio or that they have arthritis–diseases which the employer finds understandable and more acceptable. If he does get the job, the hemophiliac may be forced later on to cover up bleeding episodes and to invent excuses for frequent absences, which eventually may wear thin with the employer.

Although there was little difference between high and low severe regarding concealment, there was a wide difference between the severity groups on the frequency of being turned down for jobs. The high severe had 28 percent who had never been refused jobs for hemophilia reasons, compared with 52 percent of the low severe. The high severe had 18 percent and the low severe had only 6 percent who had been turned down seven or more times; so that the high severe had a far higher percentage who had been refused jobs and they were refused more frequently than were the low severe.

For the success-severity groups we found the following percentages who stated they had never been turned down for a job: successful low-severe, 55 percent; successful high-severe, 37 percent; unsuccessful low-severe, 35 percent; unsuccessful high-severe, 13 percent. Clearly, severity is an important factor in employer refusal; however, the difference between the two high-severe and the two low-severe groups and the similarity between the successful high and the unsuccessful low indicate that other factors are also involved.

Table XXV summarizes some of the above findings.

Despite the feeling held by many hemophiliacs that employers do not want to hire them and that their condition is misunderstood by employers, 93 percent of the employed and 85 percent of the unemployed said they had good relationships with their employers. Further, *respondents who revealed their hemophilia to their employer remained on those jobs for longer periods of time and had a higher percentage of good relationships with the employer.* Employers who are willing to hire hemophiliacs seem prepared to accept some absenteeism and other inconvenience and thus tend to be more tolerant of the problems posed by the hemophilic employee.

TABLE XXV

PATTERNS OF JOB REFUSAL
AND OF INFORMING EMPLOYER RE: HEMOPHILIA

Group	*Never Turned Down Because of Hemophilia* %	*Concealed Hemophilia from Last Employer** %
Employed	51	26
Unemployed	27	30
Low-severe	52	26
High-severe	28	23
Successful low-severe	55	25
Successful high-severe	37	22
Unsuccessful low-severe	35	33
Unsuccessful high-severe	13	15

*Excludes the never employed and self employed.

Respondents whose occupations were in the professional, executive, and managerial fields tended to reveal their condition, while those in manual labor did not. White collar and clerical workers were inconsistent, sometimes disclosing and sometimes not. These findings suggest that positions that require more responsibility, training, and education, and where the employee is judged more on merit and ability than on the need to conform to regular hours, are optimal for hemophiliacs.

In addition to answering questionnaire items in our study, more than two thirds of the respondents wrote in remarks covering various topics or personal concern.* About 150 respondents mentioned specific employment problems, many having to do with employer problems. The chief comments referred to employers' unwillingness to hire hemophiliacs, job applications turned down for hemophilia, expressions of fear of job loss because of illness or disclosure, occasions when the respondent

*See Chapter 11

had been fired when the employer learned of his hemophilia or had lowered respondent in rank and duties.

In general, those who complained about employers felt the latter were uninformed about hemophilia. As one respondent phrased it, "They look at you as if they expected you to start bleeding all over the place." While absenteeism is a real problem in hiring hemophiliacs, many hemophiliacs feel that employers refused them jobs out of ignorance and fear rather than for such practical reasons. They feel that they are unfairly stigmatized and that employers should be informed of their true capabilities and potential. Some speculated that jobs could be found where the work schedule might be flexible enough to handle occasional absences; a number of respondents said they would be willing to work extra hard to make up for lost time or that they could make up time so that time lost would not be work lost. Several respondents, in fact, stated that they consistently worked harder than their fellows in order to hold their jobs, since they felt they started out at a disadvantage. By and large, the respondents stressed that employers would not suffer losses in hiring hemophiliacs, but that it would first be necessary to break down employer resistance stemming from lack of information rather than from practical considerations.

ABSENTEEISM

The problem is not a simple one, because factors such as absenteeism and undertraining are realistic for many hemophiliacs. Not many jobs can tolerate chronic absenteeism; however, there are perhaps more kinds of work which can tolerate some absenteeism than one commonly thinks. On the other hand, not all hemophiliacs have frequent or long absences from work. Table XXVI shows the incidence of absences from work due to hemophilia for the employed and the unemployed.

This table reflects a relatively high absenteeism rate among hemophiliacs, however, it can also be seen that the majority of the employed average less than two days a month absence from work. Many hemophiliacs attend work when they are hemorrhaging, if they do not consider the hemorrhage severe. A number of respondents go to work although suffering constant pain; some have jobs which cause them steady discomfort, but they feel the necessity to continue them.

TABLE XXVI

NUMBER OF DAYS ABSENT FROM WORK PER YEAR
OF EMPLOYED AND UNEMPLOYED

Days Absent per Year	*Employed (N = 564)* %	*Unemployed (N = 152)* %
None	11	3.0
1-3 days	9	0.5
4 – 7 days	8	7.0
8 – 14 days	13	11.0
15 – 30 days	22	18.0
31 – 60 days	14	18.0
61 – + days	8	25.0
Gave two answers, unspecified	3	0.5
No answer	11	17.0
	99	99.0

Absenteeism and severity are related, with the high-severe having over 80 percent absent from work for more than fourteen days per year. The low-severe had 40 percent in that category. Information which might help employers reach a decision in hiring hemophiliacs would include information about the varying degrees of severity among hemophiliacs. Low and medium-severity hemophiliacs appear to be good job risks, if the job can tolerate a modicum of absenteeism. Lack of job training and/or education are, however, even more important for the hemophiliac than the probability of absenteeism. Those who have received adequate education and training tend to be employed, whether or not they have frequent absences from work. Some have found employers and/or jobs that tolerate absenteeism, but most have made other adjustments and have found ways to circumvent the problem such as making up time. *Many feel that self-employment is the answer and have either achieved it or are working toward that goal, e.g. in such occupations as real estate, small business, and the professions.* An important consideration is whether or not absences will interfere with the work of other employees A felicitous kind of occupation is where the hemophiliac's work is relatively independent of his fellow workers, where he can simply take up where he left off, without production suffering from his absence. Such job possibilities should be explored, with more emphasis on these requirements and less on safety—within obvious limits.

OTHER REASONS FOR JOB REFUSAL

Respondents were asked to respond to a multiple-choice question which listed various reasons for being turned down for jobs. Table XXVII lists the reasons and percentages of hemophiliacs turned down for each reason.

TABLE XXVII

REASONS RESPONDENTS WERE TURNED DOWN FOR JOBS BY EMPLOYERS

Reasons Given by Employer	*Total Sample (N = 1,055)** %	*Employed (N = 564)** %	*Unemployed (N = 152)** %
Work too strenuous, hard for hemophiliac	10	9	19.0
Dangerous working conditions for hemophiliac	11	11	18.0
Work production of hemophiliac would be low	5	5	12.0
Hemophiliac would be absent too often	18	17	37.0
Company's status with Workmen's Compensation or insurance company would be affected	14	14	24.0
No emergency facilities for hemorrhaging	4	4	10.0
Other (various not listed above)	8	0	0.7

*Respondents could list more than one reason

State workmen's compensation programs and private insurance companies were seen as hindrances by respondents who checked that alternative and who mentioned them in their later remarks. According to the respondents' reports, these agencies object to employers' hiring hemophiliacs on the basis of risk. Hemophiliacs feel that such practices discriminate against them unfairly; they are in the double jeopardy of risking serious injury, yet they have no financial protection and, indeed, are denied access to means whereby they might provide their own financial protection, by working on a job.

A few hemophiliacs said they had been able to sign waivers, absolving the company, workmen's compensation, and/or insurance companies from liability and thus had obtained jobs. Others have offered to do this but have been denied jobs anyway on the basis of risk.

OTHER OBSTACLES TO FINDING WORK FOR THE HEMOPHILIAC

Respondents were asked to reply to the question, "If you feel that hemophilia interferes with your chances for finding a job, how does it interfere? (Check one or more)." The results are shown in Table XXVIII.

TABLE XXVIII

WAYS IN WHICH HEMOPHILIA INTERFERES WITH FINDING WORK

Interferences	*Total Sample (N = 1,055)** %	*Employed (N = 564)** %	*Unemployed (N = 152)** %
Respondent feels too handicapped to work	8	5	22
Most jobs are too strenuous for hemophiliac	26	21	38
Many work situations too dangerous	23	20	31
Employers don't want to hire hemophiliac	32	31	53
Lack of previous training due to hemophilia	17	14	27
Respondent can work part-time only, and it is difficult to find part-time work	9	6	15
Respondent can work at home only	3	2	7

*Respondents could select more than one alternative.

Twenty-five percent of the entire sample (32% of the employed, 9% of the unemployed and 3% of the never employed) selected the alternative "Hemophilia does *not* interfere with finding work." Such findings tend to confirm the notion that those in the unsuccessful category emphasize the incapacitating nature of their hemophilia to a far greater degree than do the successful. It is of interest also that most hemophiliacs do not feel too handicapped to work, but rather, tend to blame employers for their employment difficulties.

PERFORMANCE AND DIFFICULTIES ON THE JOB ENCOUNTERED BY HEMOPHILIACS

Respondents' Self-rating of Job Performance

When asked to indicate the difficulties they have encountered on the job, 38 percent of the total sample(42% of the employed and only 24% of the unemployed) said "none." In addition, of 301 respondents who wrote comments at the end of the questionnaire, 29 percent said they were pleased with their performance or made other positive remarks regarding work experience; 37 percent made negative remarks regarding job performance or experience. Only 7 percent of the unemployed stated they had done well at work, while 66 percent said they had not. Of the employed, 39 percent were pleased with their job experience and 28 percent made negative remarks concerning work.

It thus appears that many hemophiliacs are dissatisfied with their work experiences, ranging from those who have a few specific complaints to those who are dissatisfied to the point of giving up.

The respondents' comments about employment were analyzed in a number of ways: how they rated their performance–whether they said they functioned well on the job or not; how the respondent felt about work, his own performance, work situation, past experiences, and work potential. There was considerable overlap in these two classifications–if a respondent said "I have a wonderful job and am doing very well on it," he would be scored as performing well and as being pleased with his work experience. Some, however, felt that while they performed well on their jobs, they did so with great difficulty or had difficulties in finding work or securing advancement in work status. These respondents were scored as performing well, but as being dissatisfied with their work experience in one way or another.

Severity was related to such self-reports of performance and feelings about work, in that fewer of the high severe than the low severe performed well and were pleased, yet the differences were not so great as might be anticipated. Of the high severe, 30 percent said they performed well, were successful, et cetera, and 38 percent indicated they were pleased with employment experiences; 16 percent said they sometimes performed well and sometimes not, depending on their health or other circumstances. Of the low severe, 48 percent said they performed well, 16 percent said they sometimes did and sometimes not, depending on health and other circumstances, and 46 percent were pleased with their work experiences. The intermediate severe with high number of major hemorrhages (but low in minor hemorrhages) had only 23 percent who were pleased with their work experiences.

Problems Encountered on the Job

Surprisingly infrequent is the problem of the hemophiliac who feels he is too handicapped to work or who would like to quit working because of his health. Only six respondents said they would like to be able to quit work, and twenty-six said they were unable to work because of health; although 105 respondents over the age of twenty-five had been unemployed for a relatively long period of time. Most of the comments expressed the idea in one way or another that the individual desired to work.

The most frequent problems encountered on the job according to 841 respondents were absenteeism (33%), too much standing up on the job (21%), working hours too long (14%), dangerous or pain-producing working conditions for hemophiliac (13%), and lack of training (7%).

Some ways in which hemophilia handicaps the respondents on the jobs are in chances for promotion (employed, 16%;

unemployed 21%); transfer to another department or duties (employed, 9%; unemployed, 13%); the amount of work respondent can do (employed, 25%; unemployed, 40%). Some said they were unable to find the kind of work they were best trained and suited for because of hemophilia; a few said they were unable to carry out such work because of hemophilia.

Special Facilities and Privileges

Despite the relatively frequent occurrence of some kind of difficulty on the job because of hemophilia, most hemophiliacs do not ask for special privileges or facilities; 78 percent of the employed and 67 percent of the unemployed did not. These percentages should be contrasted with the findings that approximately 60 percent of the employed and 76 percent of the unemployed mention one or more problems at work. Probably, most hemophiliacs attempt to compete on the general labor market and fear that special requests would antagonize employers. The most frequent kind of special privilege requested was for more sick leave than granted to other employees, 10 percent of both the employed and the unemployed selected that alternative from a list of possible privileges.

SATISFACTION WITH OCCUPATION

From the responses to two questions, it appears that most hemophiliacs would choose different occupations from the ones in which they are currently engaged. The two questions asked were (1) "What kind of job would you like to have if different from the one you have at present?" and (2) "If you did not have hemophilia, what kind of work would you like to do?" Since these were open-ended questions, the respondents could write in any vocational choice, or "same" as at present, or they could leave the question blank. Table XXIX presents the findings from these questions, the percentages being based on the number in each group who responded.

Clerical work is seen as least desirable, given the conditions in question 2, and those persons who are employed in clerical occupations infrequently reply "same" or "satisfied." Most who selected a white collar position for question 1 made a different choice in replying to question 2. The most satisfying or desirable kind of work is seen as some kind of professional or executive position. About 40 percent of the employed prefer jobs in that category; about 23 percent actually hold such jobs.

TABLE XXIX

OCCUPATIONS DESIRED BY HEMOPHILIACS

Occupation	*Employed (N = 564)*		*Unemployed (N = 152)*	
	Question 1 (N = 293)* %	*Question 2* (N = 409)* %	*Question 1* (N = 82)* %	*Question 2* (N = 111)* %
"Same" or satisfied	23	36.0	5	12.0
Professional, executive, managerial	20	18.0	18	27.0
Medical (Q, 1 only)	6	--	0	–
Out-of-door (e.g. sports, farming, forestry) (Q. 2 only)	–	15.0	–	11.0
Arts	4	3.0	13	7.0
Technical	8	6.0	12	11.0
White collar	14	6.0	13	4.0
Mechanical	4	3.0	4	10.0
Clerical	6	0.7	10	0.9
Manual labor	6	7.0	10	14.0
Other	9	4.0	15	4.0

*Number answering each question.

THE SELF-EMPLOYED

Absenteeism and Severity

Because of absenteeism and other problems associated with finding and keeping jobs many hemophiliacs feel that self-employment would be the best situation for them. One hundred four (18%) of the employed were self-employed and seventeen (11%) of the unemployed had been self-employed in their most recent position. Thus, of the 121 persons who are or were self-employed, 14 percent are currently unemployed, compared to 22 percent for the other-employed.

For several reasons it appears that absenteeism bears a strong relationship to self-employment. The index of severity showed the self-employed to have 29 percent of high severity, while the other-employed had 22 percent. Probably related to that finding is the fact that the self-employed had a greater percentage reporting a high absenteeism rate, and many commented that absenteeism was their greatest problem.

In general, hemophilia was reported more frequently to be handicapping for the self-employed. They had a higher proportion who reported that hemophilia interferes with finding work, more frequently reported difficulties on the job due to hemophilia, had a higher tendency to quit their last job, and quit school for reasons of health and to state that hemophilia prevents them from working full-time. There is, however, no difference between the groups as to whether they are actually working full-time or part-time; most in both groups work full-time.

We found that 38 percent of the self-employed and 28 percent of the other-employed had been confined to wheelchairs at some time, either in the present or in the past.

Occupations of the Self-employed

Table XXX gives the percentages of self-employed and other-employed in the various occupations listed.

The majority of the self-employed in the first occupation listed are in some kind of business. Table XXXI lists the kinds of enterprises in which these two groups of respondents are working. It is notable that the self-employed have avoided businesses involving clerical work. Small business such as secretarial services, telephone answering, bookkeeping services, and other similar enterprises, which can be done piecemeal and even in the home, do not occur to any great extent among these self-employed respondents. This supports the earlier finding that clerical work is least desirable to these respondents.

The other-employed have a relatively high percentage in industry, employed as laborers or supervisors and in white collar and clerical positions.

TABLE XXX

OCCUPATIONS OF SELF-EMPLOYED AND OTHER-EMPLOYED

Occupation	*Self-employed (N = 121)* %	*Other-employed (N = 560)** %
Professional, executive, managerial business owners	64	11
Arts	7	2
Supervisors	0	4
White collar	5	19
Technical	10	13
Clerical	1	16
Services	7	10
Skilled, semiskilled, unskilled labor	6	24
Other	0	1
	100	100

*Twenty-five cases are missing from this table.

TABLE XXXI

Enterprise	*Self-employed (N = 121)* %	*Other-employed (N = 588** %
Education	1	2
Building and construction	3	5
Transportation	5	6
Manufacturing and assembly	9	31
Government	0	11
Farming	9	3
Professional	16	7
Communications	4	4
Business	47	26
Other	5	3
Insufficient information	1	1
	100	99

*Seven cases missing.

The business category includes such businesses as retail store, advertising agency, barber shop, watch repair, automobile agency, bank, laundry and cleaning plant, motel, realty company, insurance, pharmaceuticals, dog breeding and kennels.

Some of the self-employed that are engaged in farming share

that enterprise with members of their immediate families. They were considered self-employed if they were at least part-owners of the farm. Most of the other-employed in farming are farm laborers. The respondents who own or work on farms generally have done farm work since childhood, most of them sharing in the heavy and sometimes dangerous work involved.

Income of Self-employed

The income of the self-employed seems to be no higher and may even be considerably lower than that of the other-employed. Many of the self-employed declined to answer the question regarding income; it is probable that their incomes were in the lower brackets.

TABLE XXXII

INCOME FOR SELF-EMPLOYED AND OTHER-EMPLOYED

Income	*Self-employed (N = 121)* %	*Other-employed (N = 588)** %
Under $50 per week	22	18
$50 to $75 per week	14	22
$76 to $100 per week	10	22
Over $100 per week	33	34
No information	21	4
	100	100

It seems likely that many of the self-employed have sacrificed the goal of greater income for independence, for situations where they can work according to their physical condition. They may produce less, but they are not in danger of losing their income entirely, unless their business should fail or they became totally disabled. Most hemophiliacs find their physical condition fluctuates, with good and bad periods. The self-employed have set up a situation which can cover the bad times. It should be added, however, that absenteeism and other work problems are not the only motives for becoming self-employed. Some, including those who indicate a high degree of severity, work hard and steadily whether or not they are hemorrhaging or in pain, or both. Ambition, self-development, self-expression, and the opportunity to earn a good living are as important to hemophiliacs as to anyone else, as shown by the high achievement of many of our respondents.

Summary of Vocational Situation

Four main groups were identified in our study with regard to employment status. They were the employed, the still in-school,, the unemployed, and the never-employed. Of all the respondents, 20 percent were in the last two categories and thus 80 percent were considered to be fulfilling their expected vocational roles. In addition, some of the unemployed had held their previous positions for long periods of time and/or had been only recently unemployed, and many of the never-employed were between the ages of sixteen and twenty-five years.

Occupations were found to vary in type over a wide range, from respondents in the professions, executive-managerial, and white collar positions to clerical and skilled-unskilled labor. It was found that hemophiliacs do not necessarily limit themselves to sedentary or physically nonhazardous positions and that severity of hemophilia, except at the extreme, is not related to type of occupation.

Income and stability of employment were unexpectedly high for the respondents, with the unemployed showing considerably lower income and achievement than did the employed.

Health reasons, particularly hemophilia, were the most frequent reasons given for previous or present unemployment. The unemployed were found to give this reason more frequently than the employed. Additionally, the unemployed tended to state "health" as their reason for leaving previous employment, while the employed more frequently left because they found a better job. From these and other findings it appears the unemployed stress their hemophiliac condition as a hindrance to finding and keeping employment to a greater degree than do the employed. It was also found that the unemployed, as a group, have a greater incidence of a high degree of severity than did the employed, although both groups contain high and low-severity respondents.

The overview of employment shows the majority of the respondents to be successful in their vocational situation, if gainful employment for relatively lengthy periods of time and often involving high degrees of skill, responsibility, education, and training can be considered to be criteria of success. This is a different picture of the hemophiliac from that which is generally held and is indicative of the higher potential of which this population is capable than is generally believed.

Vocational Success Versus Nonsuccess

Two groups were compared, the successful and the unsuccessful. The single criterion of success used was present employment. In order to rule out the factors of age and length of unemployment, the unsuccessful included the following: unemployed/never-employed, twenty-five years of age and over, unemployed at least seven months (N = 105). The successful were employed, twenty-five years of age and over (N= 447). The unsuccessful comprised 19 percent of the potential working force who were twenty-five years of age and over.

The most important difference between the successful and unsuccessful was in the far greater percentage of the latter in the high severity category. This difference was large enough to be considered partially accountable for the extreme differences found between the groups in their employment and social and personal characteristics. The unsuccessful were much lower in every respect on the employment variables, had a lower educational achievment, and had received more financial aid. The unsuccessful included fewer who were married and if married had a lower tendency to have children. From self-report they appear to be less active in their daily lives than are the successful.

From the standpoint of an overall view of the employment and the social and personal variables under study, the unsuccessful low-severity group appear to be the most "unsuccessful" of the four groups. They tended to emphasize their physical disability to a greater extent, were least active, had the lowest tendency to have children if married, the lowest educational achievement, and the lowest vocational achievement. This group of men appear to represent the hemophiliac who has "given up." This pattern appears to have emerged at an early age and was most detectable in their tendency to quit school because of health, despite their lower severity rating than that of two of the other groups. While the sample size is small for this group (26), for the purposes of generalization, there is little doubt they represent a larger population, many of whom were not picked up in the analysis because of the data analysis operations involved in this study. It is probable, however, that this group is least numerous in the overall hemophiliac population. It is these men who should be most detectable at an early age on whom special rehabilitation efforts should be concentrated, particularly in the areas of education, attitudes, and social development. They are probably more hampered by their attitudes toward their hemophilic condition than by their actual physical condition. The unsuccessful highs, on the other hand, present a different kind of rehabilitation problem, although in general they tend to take a more negative view of their situation than do the successful groups. Their attitudes have, perhaps, more basis in reality in that their experiences with regard to their physical condition have contained a greater amount and intensity of physical trauma.

The successful high-severity group, by contrast, appear to be men who have attempted to overcome, ignore, and play down their physical disability. They have placed more emphasis on achievement, beginning at an early age in school, and have attempted to lead more nearly normal lives despite their "objective" appearance of greater physical handicap. A glance at Tables XX and XXIV will show their occupational level to be relatively high, their level of income to be good, and a tendency to show a great deal of stability in their work picture.

The differences between these groups, then, is probably representative of some of the various ways in which hemophiliacs adapt to their condition. More should be learned about the ways in which the successful highs have gone about achieving their adaptation, and the same is true for the unsuccessful lows. Such findings could have ramifications for other physically handicapped groups in terms of rehabilitation efforts and early detection of symptoms of maladjustment.

Special Conditions, Problems in Relation to Work

According to the findings of the respondents in this sample, hemophiliacs receive very little professional aid in finding work, but rather, locate jobs either by job hunting or through personal contacts such as relatives and friends.

The two major problems for hemophiliacs in finding jobs are poor preparation for work in terms of education and training, and employer discrimination. Those hemophiliacs who are well educated and/or trained for jobs do tend to find employment. Most hemophiliacs have been turned down for jobs by employers because of hemophilia with the result that many of the respondents withhold their condition from prospective employers. Such withholding appears to create further problems for some hemophiliacs, in that concealment often leads to anxiety and guilt and periods of absenteeism are difficult to explain to the employer. Thus, while concealment may aid in obtaining a job, it may also contribute to losing it.

Many respondents expressed the idea that employers discriminate against them more as the result of ignorance of the true ramifications of hemophilia and the actual potential of the hemophiliac, than as a result of actual knowledge. Most hemophiliacs feel they are more capable of vocational achievement than they are given credit for by employers, and by the general public, and that they are capable of more achievement than their opportunities have permitted. They also feel they are less of a risk, in terms of bodily injury, than is popularly believed and many prefer nonsedentary jobs even including an element of physical risk. There appears to be some relationship between employer-refusal and severity, the successful low-severe having been refused least frequently. The unsuccessful have a far higher percentage of refusal than do the successful.

With regard to keeping jobs, the main problem for hemophiliacs is absenteeism, although about 42 percent of the employed have relatively few absences per year. The unemployed have only about 20 percent in that category. Absenteeism and severity have a strong positive relationship.

Some hemophiliacs stated they work harder than other employees in order to compensate for any deficiencies and to combat employer attitudes. Some have arranged situations whereby they are able to make up work lost because of absenteeism Some work under conditions of severe pain and moderate hemorrhaging in order to keep their jobs.

One frequent complaint was that workmen's compensation and insurance companies refuse to endorse hemophiliacs' employment, so employers refuse to hire them for that reason. This was found to be the case even when the hemophiliac offered to waive such benefits in order to get the job.

It should be pointed out, however, that the majority of hemophiliacs, especially the unemployed and the never-employed, feel that hemophilia, as a disease, does present problems in finding and keeping jobs.

In terms of job satisfaction, satisfaction with own performance, and with work experiences, it appears that about one third of the respondents are satisfied or have had good work experiences and about one third feel they have performed poorly, and are dissatisfied. The employed showed a far greater percentage who were pleased with their work experiences and performance than did the unemployed. Severity was related to reported performance and satisfaction, with the low severe reporting more positive experiences and attitudes. The high severe, however, had 30 percent who felt they were successful in their work performance and 38 percent who indicated they were pleased with their work experiences. It can be seen that severity and reported work experience are less related than are work experience and success-nonsuccess. Most respondents indicated they would prefer work other than that in which they are engaged, although about 36 percent of the employed would select the same work as at present.

Perhaps the most important conclusion to be drawn from these findings is that, while there are very real problems associated with hemophilia and employment, most hemophiliacs feel capable of work and of greater achievement than their opportunities have offered. Most hemophiliacs apparently attempt to achieve on the labor market in the same manner as do nonhemophiliacs and with striving many have accomplished this goal, some despite severe physical handicaps. It seems safe to say that most hemophiliacs would agree that their society presents barriers to vocational success in at least the same magnitude as does their physical condition.

The Self-employed

Because of the problems of absenteeism and employer discrimination, many hemophiliacs feel that self-employment is the best solution. Our study included 121 respondents who were self-employed.

This group showed a lower unemployment rate but a higher absenteeism and severity rating. They also found hemophilia to present more of a hindrance in their work than did the other-employed.

The results seem to indicate that income for the self-employed may be lower than for the other-employed.

Chapter 8

EMPLOYMENT: SOME GENERAL CONSIDERATIONS

AFTER the review of employment conditions and characteristics in the two preceding chapters, it is timely to consider some broad social trends and factors that are influencing the employment situation today, and can be expected to grow in importance in the future.

A revision in the nature of work and occupations, which may have relevance to the problems of hemophiliacs, is occurring in the United States. The economist Dr. Eli Ginzberg has pointed out that the occupational picture in the United States is changing in that this country now has essentially a service economy(10). Two out of every three workers are now providing services rather than producing goods. Such physically demanding occupations as agriculture, manufacturing, mining, and construction now account for only one out of three workers. Projections for the future indicate that if the present rate of technological development continues, there will be only one worker needed in production for every ten in the services by the year 2000.

There are some important consequences from the shift in the United States to a service economy. First, services tend to use and hire trained people so that the question of access to education and training becomes crucial; education is the determinant, the path along which one acquires skills. Other things being equal, the more education a person has initially, the more likely he is to be successful and to remain in the field which he enters.

This changing character of the economy has implications for hemophiliacs which are both positive and negative. The first implication is clearly that physically demanding occupations will no longer be of as much significance; the possible dangers to hemophiliacs in undertaking factory work, farm work, construction work will diminish, and there will be many alternatives they can turn to. Even as recently as five years ago, when we conducted our study, fully 40 percent of employed or recently employed hemophiliacs were in unskilled or skilled positions, of a nature that demanded physical exertion and that therefore had the drawbacks of physical labor for hemophiliacs.

The question of education for the new professions and technical fields available becomes crucially important. Hemophiliacs should thus be assisted and encouraged to remain in school as long as possible for preparation for the newer fields. What this will require in terms of working with the educational system, of special provisions for early counseling and guidance will be discussed at a later point. But we can be clear that the future of hemophiliacs vocationally lies in attaining a high standard of education for the technical, professional, and service fields.

There is a particular area in the service spectrum which should be stressed, what can be called the human services. This term refers to positions in the various aspects of health care, social welfare, rehabilitation counseling, mental health education, et cetera. In the United States and elsewhere, there is a distinct movement to increase the supplies of persons recruited for these fields; because many developing social programs having to do with the poor, ghetto dwellers, racial minorities and the underprivileged require additional cadres of such professional personnel. There is also a developing effort in the United States to re-think and revise the requirements for professional certification in the fields of health, social welfare, and mental health. The purpose is to establish categories of jobs which can be handled by persons with less than a full professional training, e.g. medical assistants, social-work aides, mental health assistants.

The writer would contend that this general area of the human services offers an attractive and suitable employment field for many hemophiliacs. Not only are the positions not physically demanding, but they involve close contact with people, socializing experience which in and of itself has values for persons with a disability, who may have experienced some social isolation in growing up. Persons who have grown up under the limitations of a chronic condition may acquire a greater sensitivity to the problems of others and a greater ability to empathize with other persons having social or physical disabilities.

As we have seen in the previous chapters, hemophiliacs are capable of a more effective vocational adaptation than had been believed in the past. In our study, it was found that three quarters of the hemophiliacs were working in a wide spectrum of occupations.

Other recent studies of hemophiliacs have shown similar findings. Bronks and Blackburn in Sheffield, England, found that 77 percent of the ninety patients they were following who had left school, were working at the time that their survey was made(3). More than 65 percent of hemophiliacs classified as having severe symptoms had been at work for more than 60 percent of the last five years. Patients less severely involved with milder hemophilia had correspondingly better records of steady employment. The vast majority of the patients followed by Bronks and Blackburn had been educated in regular English schools, not special schools for the physically handicapped. In Los Angeles, a follow-up study at the Orthopedic Hospital reports that about 70 percent of hemophiliacs of working age were employed in April, 1967, with another 10 percent being trained for work by the State Vocational Rehabilitation Agency. (Information supplied by Mrs. Charlotte Taylor, Rehabilitation Counselor, Orthopedic Hospital, Los Angeles.)

While the ability of the hemophiliacs to work is well established, there are some limiting factors; an important one is employer attitudes and employer education. As noted, our study found that the two major problems for hemophiliacs in finding jobs were poor preparation in terms of education and training, and employer discrimination. Most hemophiliacs believe that employers discriminate against them out of ignorance of the true problems of hemophiliacs and of their actual potential. Most hemophiliacs feel they are more capable of vocational adjustment than they are given credit for by employers and the general public. They also feel they are less of a risk in terms of body injury than is popularly believed. Certainly, in the United States, employer discrimination and employer attitudes have some connection with the problems of insurance and workmen's compensation. It is interesting to contrast the situation in England with that in the United States, because the British have innovated a social measure which holds wide promise; whereas the United States is still relying on educational processes with employers and on the latter's good will. In 1944, probably as a result of wartime manpower shortages, legislation was passed in England which required that each establishment employing twenty or more persons have a minimum of 5 percent of handicapped employees. In order to qualify for placement, handicapped individuals go on a national registry, and special counselors place such employees when they need assistance in finding work. This system has worked very well for all categories of physically and mentally handicapped in the United Kingdom; the writer has been surprised for sometime how little is known of it in our own country. In the United States the experience and the education of employers as to the potential abilities of persons with chronic disabilities would be greatly strengthened by such legislation.

It would seem quite possible to reduce the 25 percent of the unemployed in our study to a "hard core" figure of 10 percent or less, through the combination of such legislation and some other specific social provisions which will be discussed later.

Just as a rather broad social trend was mentioned at the beginning of this chapter, so it is useful to close with one. Every thoughtful person is aware of a worldwide rebellion on the part of young people. The writer believes this has many healthy and positive aspects, but whether or not one agrees with all the actions and ideas of young people these days, it is nevertheless necessary to understand that this revolution is probably irreversible. What this means is that parents cannot and should not try to dictate to their children with regard to such important matters as the choice of an occupation and life style. Parents can suggest, they can set an example, they can make choices possible, but the basic decision needs to be made by the young person himself. This is as true in the choice of a lifelong occupation as in the choice of a lifelong marital partner. Sometimes, it is hard to apply this in our own families, but the writer is persuaded that the greatest benefit for the greatest number will result from our doing so. Perhaps the temptation to make a decision or to force a decision is greater when parents know their child has a chronic disability. But it is certain that hemophilic youngsters, like the physically normal, should and will make their own choices.

Chapter 9

VOCATIONAL COUNSELING AND PLACEMENT

FROM the foregoing sections of this book the dimensions of the vocational problems facing hemophiliacs have become clearer.

Vocational success can be viewed as a product of the interaction of adequate educational preparation, suitable choice of a career or occupation, and existing job opportunities. Without the presence of all three elements in the equation, frustration and difficulties in this major area of living are highly probable, if not unavoidable.

With the hemophilic child, as we have seen, educational deficits and deprivation are common. Of equal importance is the deprivation of social and environmental experience which can result from hemophilia-imposed isolation. Rusalem has well-stated the effects of such deprivation on vocational choices:

> Hospital and homebound children who fail to observe a variety of occupations in action in the community tend to narrow their vocational choices prematurely, and to have a higher incidence of inappropriate occupational choices than other children. Similarly, adolescents who for any reason fail to have remunerative work experiences in conjunction with school and home life tend to manifest symptoms of retarded vocational development(16).

A close coordination between medical care and educational, vocational, and parent counseling programs which emphasize rounded social experience wherever possible can thus help steer and prepare hemophiliacs toward suitable and satisfying vocational choices. In the first instance, one would like to see the public vocational authorities take responsibility for enlarging the scope of their services in order to bring this improved coordination about.

Made several years ago, our own study indicated that only 12 percent of hemophiliacs had had any contacts with their state division of vocational rehabilitation. These state agencies–jointly financed by federal and state funds—have the basic responsibility of providing both physical restoration and vocational training or retraining for physically disabled persons of working age and potential. The Federal-State Vocational Rehabilitation program is one of the oldest and best-established social service and medical programs in the country, and it could have been expected to help many hemophiliacs prepare for a suitable occupation.

The small percentage of hemophiliacs in our study who were actually helped by this source was puzzling and surprising. But explanations are not hard to find. First, like many federal-state service programs, (and unlike the Veteran's Administration) discretion as to what categories of the disabled are included for aid is left up to the states; and state programs in this regard are usually guided by their own medical consultants. From caution, prudence, or simple lack of acquaintance with hemophiliacs, some state consultants simply were unaware of the true needs and potentials of hemophiliacs, assuming that if they were relatively well, the latter needed no assistance; while if their hemophilic involvements were severe, they were too risky or otherwise unfeasible for rehabilitation.

Secondly, many hemophiliacs were simply unaware of the services of DVR agencies; or if aware, were reluctant to apply to them for fear of the stigma of "charity," or of becoming entangled in bureaucratic red tape. These subjective factors should probably be viewed as an example of the general and regrettable lack of knowledge of and contact with helpful community sources that has characterized many hemophiliacs in the past.

Fortunately, this unawareness and isolation from potential help is changing. With the growth of knowledge of hemophilia among medical care, rehabilitation, and social service agencies, often stimulated by the educational programs and lobbying of the National Hemophilia Foundation, there is today a much wider and sounder knowledge and more utilization of community resources. The state divisions of rehabilitation have become more knowledgeable and accepting of hemophiliacs as applicants for service, partly as a result of the activities of the work of headquarters staff in Washington, partly through rather wide circulation of our own study to the staffs of the state divisions, and partly from the several training institutes for rehabilitation counselors, nurses, and teachers organized by the National Hemophilia Foundation and by other groups.

In addition, in the past few years, the National Hemophilia Foundation has conducted a series of behavioral science evaluation centers in various cities, at which university and other personnel in rehabilitation counseling, social work, psychiatry, and other professional fields have evaluated and counseled teen-age hemophiliacs and their parents on life problems with an emphasis on vocations.

Experience in such seminars has convinced the Foundation of the importance of early social experience for hemophilic boys, along lines that we have previously discussed, and of the indispensability of early prevocational counseling.

On behalf of the Foundation, Rusalem(16) suggests that the following provisions are important in influencing vocational preparation.

1. Since vocational development is interwoven with total psychosocial development, families with a hemophilic child should receive early and consistent family counseling, social casework, and, if needed, psychiatric treatment.
2. Parents should be encouraged by public health nurses, visiting counselors, and, most important of all, physicians to take sensible risks in relation to their children and expose them to as many normal life experiences as possible.
3. Special educators working with hemophilic children should make efforts to provide these children with compensatory educational activities of a vocationally significant nature wherever experience deprivation appears to be constricting a child's development.
4. Starting at age ten and annually thereafter, each hemophilic child should be evaluated by an interdisciplinary team with provisions being made for early follow-up so that the team recommendations can be implemented without delay.
5. National, regional, or state vocational development centers for hemophilic secondary school students should be established through which these young people may obtain the needed vocational services that are usually denied to them.
6. Educators, guidance personnel, and rehabilitation counselors should be provided with information concerning hemophilia and help in understanding how they function most effectively with hemophilic students.
7. Finally, parents should be helped to understand why professional

intervention is almost universally needed in the vocational adjustment of the hemophilic student and they should be prepared by caseworkers and counselors to seek out and accept such help at critical points in the child's development.

In the writer's opinion, these recommendations, if adopted, would go far to overcome many of the potentially disabling aspects of the hemophilic boy's social and educational development. The truncation of growth-producing, maturing experiences that results from enforced absences from school, and reduced opportunities for social interaction, can be compensated for by planned provisions at the most "critical points in the child's development."

Who would sponsor and provide such services is of course a moot point. Some of the recommendations in Chapter 12 are addressed to it. It is sufficient to indicate that a partnership between public and voluntary effort in this field is both desirable and feasible.

Family counseling, social casework, psychiatric treatment as needed, should ideally be made available to hemophiliacs and their families by community agencies, public or voluntary, that are already offering such services to the general public.

The National Hemophilia Foundation and its Chapters should continue to have a strong role in educating other professionals–in the schools, medical care agencies, private medical practise, public employment and vocational agencies–employers and trade unions as to the special characteristics, needs and potentials of hemophiliacs. As a voluntary body, able to move quickly, it is also in a position to inaugurate small pilot programs, innovations in methods of social care–group counseling, parent education, vocational choice seminars, and the like. It is also uniquely equipped to sponsor some research into the determinants of vocational success, the effectiveness of various forms of social and vocational preparation, and so on.

The Foundation's interest in contributing to knowledge that will aid hemophiliacs is not in question, but its resources are limited. It would thus seem highly desirable that some of the valuable demonstrations already pioneered by the Foundation be incorporated in on-going public programs, freeing the Foundation to engage in newer studies and demonstrations in the vocational and related fields.

Chapter 10

ON BEING A CITIZEN: THE SOCIAL PARTICIPATION OF HEMOPHILIACS

WHEN one examines the situation of hemophiliacs over the past thirty years in the United States, it is apparent that there have been notable improvements.

First, they are living longer, fuller, and more normal lives—thanks chiefly to medical advances, especially in the areas of blood coagulation, transfusion, and orthopedics. Their life expectancy now approaches the normal; many are unhandicapped; most, as we have seen, hold jobs, support their families, and go about their daily business less troubled by the Damoclean sword of an earlier day.

Secondly, many hemophiliacs are receiving a more complete education than was available in the past. What is responsible for these changes and for the alteration in public attitudes that has apparently occurred?

For the latter accomplishment, the National Hemophilia Foundation—the self-help group of hemophiliacs and their relatives—must be given the largest share of credit.

Founded in 1948, the Foundation had a comparatively slow growth until the mid-1950's, when a number of prominent businessmen and professionals became interested in helping hemophiliacs. They instituted professional fund-raising and organizational campaigns that resulted in the Foundation's acquiring some four thousand members in more than forty localities, including Hawaii. Professional meetings have been organized that gave instruction and information to professionals such as teachers, social workers, and rehabilitation counselors who had largely been uninformed regarding the problems of hemophiliacs. An active counterpart, the Canadian Hemophilia Association, performs similar services in all the Canadian provinces.

Simultaneously, an international body, the World Federation of

Hemophilia Societies, was organized; it has held several international symposia on scientific subjects and has exchanged ideas and programs for hemophilia sufferers in several countries.

Hemophilia is more visibly on the map of the public's and professionals' consciousness today than ever before. The communications media often highlight hemophiliacs' problems or such medical advances as the preparation of cryoprecipitate blood fraction, by Dr. Judith Pool of Stanford. A recent best seller was a book on the Romanoffs, which devoted much attention to the role of hemophilia in their lives.

On a governmental level, various branches of the Department of Health, Education and Welfare, in Washington, have given increasing support to investigations of hemophilia, ranging from the basic study of coagulation and its defects, through medical management and orthopedic care, and, in the last five years, extending to studies of psychological and social aspects. The results of these researches frequently pay off in terms of better care and better lives for hemophiliacs.

That this growth in public understanding and professional interest should have resulted from the activities of a self-help group that was started by concerned parent-volunteers is not surprising. In an early paper, published in 1959, the writer called attention to benefits that accrued to parents from such activities.

> Like other groups of the specially disadvantaged and handicapped, hemophiliacs and their families can draw great strength from group associations. In those communities where the voluntary agency concerned with their problem exists, these families have been able to work out generally superior arrangements for blood procurement, medical services, and special schooling. The less tangible advantages of participation in such self-help groups are also worth stating. Among these are (1) overcoming the sense of isolation and overwhelming distress, frequently experienced by parents as a first reaction to the diagnosis of hemophilia; (2) provision of accurate information regarding the problems of medical management, child care, blood procurement, and so forth; (3) socialization through contacts and exchange of experience with other families who can contribute to knowledge about developmental phases and problems that can be anticipated; (4) provision of organized or informal opportunities to discuss the parents' fears, frustrations, and satisfactions arising from the particular difficulties of caring for a hemophilic child; (5)

opportunity to discuss broader and longer-range problems that can be anticipated on behalf of the child so that planning can be done; (6) possibility of securing through group action better facilities of a therapeutic and educational nature for their children; (7) cathartic effects of such personal participation, which helps to relieve anxieties by channeling them into constructive outlets(12).

This analysis followed the general lines of an earlier study made by the writer, and incorporated in a book, *Parents of the Handicapped* (Charles C Thomas, Publisher, 1961) and other publications. Readers interested in some general aspects of the origin and development of self-organized or self-help groups in the health and welfare field, in their likenesses and differences from conventionally organized social agencies, in their relationships with professionals, and their probable future, are referred to these publications.

A major index, then, of the citizen participation of hemophiliacs might be found in the degree of their activity or inactivity in the hemophilia associations. Here, our own study was not very informative, nor do we know of others that entitle us to say that participation in the self-help groups in and of itself is beneficial. We suspect that this is true, but it is also clear that only a minority of hemophiliacs take a really active part in their local group. From the comments quoted in earlier chapters, and known information about other disabled people, it is clear that some hemophiliacs prefer not to associate with other sufferers but seek their social life in the general community. Hemophiliacs who bear no physical mark of their disorder can do so more easily than such physically handicapped persons as the cerebral palsied, deaf, post-polios, and so forth.

Another way of looking at the social participation of hemophiliacs is by studying their patterns of recreation and hobbies, leisure time and friendships. Here our study did produce some detailed and relevent data, indicating that many hemophiliacs have a well-rounded personal life, and that the majority, at the least, have hobbies and regular ways of spending their leisure.

Table XXXIII presents details regarding participation in social clubs, hobbies, and other organizations.

As an indication of nonfamilial social interactions, questions were asked about the number of close friends that they had.

TABLE XXXIII

PARTICIPATION IN CLUBS, HOBBIES
N = 1,055

	Social Clubs		*Hobbies*		*Service Organizations*		*Unions*	
	No.	*%*	*No.*	*%*	*No.*	*%*	*No.*	*%*
Participate	263	24.93	831	78.77	219	20.76	239	22.65
Don't participate	686	65.02	173	16.40	679	64.36	702	66.54
No information	106	10.05	51	4.83	157	14.88	114	10.81
		100.00		100.00		100.00		100.00

Only thirty-two respondents said that they had no close friends, but one hundred did not respond to the question. Most said that they have close friends ranging in number from one or two to over twenty-six. About 17 percent said they had from three to six friends and 42 percent had seven or more friends. Some said "many" or "a few." The definition of "close friend" seems to have varied among the respondents in view of the broad range of number and the fact that it is hard to envisage having over seventeen "close" friends, although 176 respondents said that they did. It would be useful to determine further the amounts and kinds of contacts hemophiliacs have with those termed "friends." The reported number of friendships had no relation to other variables under study.

Hemophiliacs were also asked about the number of friends they had who have hemophilia or some other physical handicap. Over 65 percent said they had none; 15 percent said one or two. The rest reported higher numbers or said "several," "few," et cetera, and 9 percent gave no reply.

From these scant data it appears that many hemophiliacs seek and relate to friends in similar fashion as the nonhandicapped population, but further investigation of this point would be desirable.

LEISURE-TIME ACTIVITIES

Another question was "What are your favorite leisure-time

activities?" The responses were rated on three dimensions: (1) number of activities listed, (2) the activity level, on a scale from sedentary to strenuous, and (3) the degree of social interaction judged to be inherent in the activities.

A popular, often erroneous, picture of the hemophiliac is that he is fragile, sedentary, and socially withdrawn. Some believe that hemophiliacs should be "wrapped in cotton" and kept in an inactive state. Despite many pressures on them in that direction from parents and others, our study indicated that most of the men engage in moderate to very active leisure-time activities. They ranged from activities which are sedentary with minimal degree of active participation, to activities which require physical exertion and risk of injury. Examples from and frequency of occurrence are listed in Table XXXIV.

TABLE XXXIV

LEISURE-TIME ACTIVITIES–ACTIVITY LEVEL
N = 946

Activity Level	*Number*	*Percent*
1. Sedentary–minimal participation, e.g. reading, television, movies	112	11.8
2. Sedentary–more active participation, e.g. letter writing, table games	97	10.3
3. Combinations–preponderance of sedentary with some non- or moderate-strenuous	194	20.5
4. Nonstrenuous–e.g. Ham radio, driving auto, photography, tinkering	144	15.2
5. Light-moderate strenuous–e.g. woodworking, dancing, gardening	92	9.7
6. Combinations–preponderance of strenuous with some sedentary and nonstrenuous	168	17.8
7. Strenuous activity–e.g. boating, hunting, and fishing, tennis, football, skiing	139	14.7
	946	100.0

The idea that hemophiliacs are an inactive population is inaccurate according to the findings presented in these two tables. Table XXXIV indicates that 32 percent engage in strenuous activities (6 and 7) while 22 percent confine themselves to sedentary activities (1 and 2). Further, the non-to-moderate strenuous activities can certainly be considered active, in terms of the degree of participation required.

It is thus of considerable interest that hemophiliacs engage in rough and even dangerous sports, and that doing so is not confined to those who have less severe physical involvement. Of the most severe, 26 percent said they engaged in activities listed under 6 and 7 in Table XXXIV. It is true, of course, that the least severe had a higher percentage (37%) in those categories. Table XXXV presents comparisons between the low and the high-severe groups on activity level.

TABLE XXXV

SEVERITY OF HEMOPHILIA AND ACTIVITY LEVEL

Activity Level		*Low Severity*	*Per cent*	*High Severity*	*Per cent*
1. and 2.	Sedentary	77	21.04	49	20.94
3.	Combinations	63	17.21	64	27.35
4.	Nonstrenuous	48	13.12	36	15.39
5.	Moderate-strenuous	41	11.20	23	9.83
6. and 7.	Strenuous	137	37.43	62	26.50
		366	100.00	234	100.00

As a measure of the degree of social interaction involved in the leisure-time activities, a five-point ordinal scale was used. We judged whether or not social interaction seemed inherent in the activity and rated it accordingly. At one end of the scale were those activities which seem to require no other participant and at the other were activities which generally include at least one other participant. The middle of the scale, mixed activities, could be done alone *or* with others and included responses listing both solitary and group activities in equal proportion.

Table XXXVI illustrates data on this five-point scale and the kinds of activities in each category.

If the method used yielded accurate results, then it appears that solitary activities do predominate over group activities. Forty-five percent are in the solitary end of the scale, while 25 percent are in the group end. How these responses would compare to those of a different population remains unknown, but we find the unemployed hemophiliacs had a greater predominance of solitary activities (51%), as did the never-employed (49%), when compared to the employed (43%). The high-severe group had a slight tendency to more solitary and fewer group activities than did the low-severe group, but the difference is not statistically significant. The importance of this finding is that it indicates that the higher severity of the unemployed and never-employed does not account for their tendency to be more solitary. Age appears to be a factor, since the younger men tended to have more group activities.

TABLE XXXVI

DEGREE OF SOCIAL INTERACTION
AS JUDGED FROM LEISURE-TIME ACTIVITIES
N = 946

	Number	*Per cent*
1. *Solitary*—e.g. radio and television repair, gardening, electronics, reading	233	24.6
2. *Predominantly solitary*—e.g. car repair, playing musical instruments, photography	194	20.5
3. *Mixed*—e.g. fishing, hunting, traveling (mixed activities) or fishing and photography, bowling and reading (mixed responses)	280	29.6
4. *Predominance of group activity with some solitary*	141	14.9
5. *Group activities*—no solitary listed, e.g. dating, visiting, clubs, pool, tennis, table games	98	10.4
	946	100.0

SUMMARY

In the immediate past, many hemophiliacs did not survive, but with medical advances, survival into middle and old age is predictable for most hemophiliacs. Many hemophiliacs marry, have children, are steadily employed, and function in independent social roles.

Some hemophiliacs are chronically disabled in the sociopsychological sense, whatever the nature of their physical condition. These persons are dependent materially and socially and present problems to themselves, their families, and society. Special efforts at rehabilitation might well be directed toward them.

A broad range of educational achievement was found in the sample, from respondents with no formal education to those who have completed university work and advanced degrees. A high percentage of the sample, however, were low educational achievers who did not complete high school. The educational level achieved bears a direct relationship to occupational and personal adjustment.

Many hemophiliacs participate in active and even possibly hazardous leisure-time activities. Thus, our data indicate that hemophiliacs desire and are capable of a higher activity level than is generally assumed.

Chapter 11

HOW HEMOPHILIACS VIEW THEMSELVES AND THE WORLD

IN preceding chapters we have presented materials from our detailed study, which were based on responses to objective questions, mostly multiple choice and "yes"-"no." The questionnaire was lengthy, and to complete it was time-consuming; some items required recall of dates and facts or judgments about the past. It was surprising, therefore, to find that over two-thirds of the respondents wrote answers to the final question, which was "Please add any comments you wish to make about your situation as a hemophiliac."

Several points were notable about the written comments: (1) They were lengthy—22 percent contained over seventy-five words; 10 percent were two pages and more in length. (2) They often clarified previous responses or provided further information. (3) Many comments expressed strong feelings, positive as well as negative, about the topics mentioned; they could be classified into a limited number of categories, indicating some commonality or universality of observations and attitudes among these hemophiliacs.

This led us to the belief that valuable information was contained in these written remarks. The recurrent topics seemed representative of the most important concerns of hemophiliacs, and therefore could provide further insight into the general problems of hemophiliacs, especially the psychosocial aspects.

The main topics of the comments were classified as Advice to Parents, Employment, Education, Attitudes of Society and Groups and Organizations, Physical Aspects and Self-view, Coping Mechanisms, Attitudes toward Hemophilia. Examples of the comments in each category are presented in this chapter so that the reader may more fully grasp the distinctive tone, meaning, and mode of expression of these hemophiliacs and get a firsthand picture of their reactions to their experience, and their views of the world.

ADVICE TO PARENTS

A key question asked of respondents was, What advice would you give to parents whose child had hemophilia? It was thought this question would provide (1) direct information regarding hemophiliacs' views of child-rearing practices as they had experienced them, and (2) indirect information regarding their views of desirable parental behavior.

Sixty-nine (69%) of the respondents wrote in answers to this question, which could be classified as follows in order of greatest frequency.

Normality

This was the most frequently offered advice, and expressed the idea that the hemophilic child should be premitted great freedom of activity with few or no restrictions on his behavior.

Goals

Many hemophiliacs felt that active participation or achievement in school, in vocational, social and other activities should be encouraged by parents, and that the child should be especially encouraged to strive toward a worthwhile vocation.

Emotions and Attitudes

Many stressed the possibility of psychological damage to the child, which might occur because of the restrictions placed upon him through social isolation, setbacks in his attempts to strive, and so forth. Others were concerned with the development of healthy, or constructive or realistic attitudes toward hemophilia in order to avoid emotional problems.

Restriction of Child's Activities

Some stressed restriction of activity and careful supervision in order to prevent bodily harm to the hemophilic child. These responses were in contrast to those designated as "normality" above, and were of relatively low frequency.

Social Needs

A few emphasized the social development of the child, the importance of his achieving social skills, of having good peer-group relationships, the need for friends.

Table XXXVII shows the distribution of advice comments according to the various occupational categories mentioned in Chapter 6. Percentages are given for the entire sample and for the main occupational groups.

TABLE XXXVII

ADVICE TO PARENTS OF A HEMOPHILIC CHILD–EMPLOYMENT GROUPS

	Occupational Group				
Advice	*Total Sample (N = 732)** %	*Employed (N = 426)* %	*Unemployed (N = 106)* %	*Never Employed (N = 27)* %	*Still in School (N = 173)* %
Normality	53	51	39	33	72
Goals	32	33	45	19	24
Emotions, attitudes	26	27	19	26	29
Medical	21	22	18	26	19
Restrictions	15	15	14	26	12
Social development	5	4	5	5	8
Per cent responding	69	76	70	45	62

*Numbers are number responding to the question.

There are some noticeable differences between the groups in their recommendations for hemophilic children. The unemployed and never-employed urged a normal way of life far less frequently than the other two groups. The never-employed were concerned with medical advice to a great extent, and most often recommended restricting and protecting the child. The unemployed had the highest concern for goals and achievement. The never-employed placed least emphasis on goals in comparison with the other groups, probably reflecting the fact that they lead more sheltered and inactive lives and show greater psychological handicap as the result of hemophilia. Few of the never-employed responded to the question, which might be considered as further evidence of their greater passivity, noted in earlier chapters. The unemployed, on the other hand, show the highest concern for goals, which may reflect their feelings of frustration concerning vocational achievement.

Normality

Some representative examples of the remarks classified under "normality" follow. Many respondents recommended the avoidance of any limitations, stating that the child will learn to set his own.

> . . . If the child wants to play, use a knife or axe . . . let it. The child will have to learn the correct way of using these items. (Age 27, dairyman)

> Try to send the child to a regular school or at least simulate a normal environment as closely as possible. The physical risks are justified by the resulting mental and emotional development. (Age 17, still in school)

> Let the child live as near to an active normal life as he can. Do not be over protective. I would rather live a full normal short life than a long one not being able to do much. (Age 34, sales representative)

Some respondents who recommended "normality" believed there are reasonable or necessary limits, or unavoidable precautions, as for example:

> In my opinion, my parents managed my brother (who was also a hemophiliac) and me in a very sensible manner which, in my opinion, is one of the main reasons why I am 49 and why my brother lived to 43. We were allowed to play as we chose (within reason) with a word of caution here and there, but never in a tone that would give us a complex. We were never given the impression that we were fragile. We

were not babied. If we done something wrong, we were not spanked, but we were punished the same as my older brother and younger sister who were not afflicted. We were not carried around on a pillow like some hemophiliacs I've heard about. I believe this was a great boost mentally. (Age 49, motel owner)

Recognize his problem and help *him* to become adjusted to it. This does not mean "sheltering" him throughout his growing period, but rather educating him as to the responsibility he will have to watch out for himself when he becomes a mature adult. A certain amount of protection will be required of course, but special schools and teacher are probably unnecessary except in a small number of cases. (Age 20, out of school, never employed)

The comments stressing normality were by far the most numerous; 53 percent of the entire sample gave that advice, compared with only 15 percent who recommended restricting the child. This is one respect in which hemophiliacs' views of their situation differ from popular belief. *The majority of hemophiliacs do not want to be sheltered, and desire to take their place in society in a normal fashion.* This is true of the adults who strive to be breadwinners in the family and of adolescents who desire to be normal members of their peer group. Resistance and resentment to overprotection were frequently expressed; some rebelled at restrictions even though this could lead to injury.

Would like not to be cautioned all the time to be careful. Have always resented not being allowed to take part in sports. Did it anyway. Most of the time I got hurt playing sports. I have reached the age now, where I realize the danger. I have a limitation in my right arm because of bleedings and I also have a short leg because of a hip injury. (Age 17, still in school)

Approximately 10 percent of the respondents expressed attitudes toward their own parents in the comments or in answering the "advice" question. The negative remarks about parents generally referred to overprotection, overemphasis on disability, and de-emphasis on achievement, by parents. The positive remarks appreciated parents who encouraged independence and striving and who had provided a nonrestrictive environment. Some respondents, in fact, reported a pattern of concealing injury from their parents in order to avoid recriminations and restrictions.

I have been particularly fortunate in having parents who believe

> that anything can be accomplished if one wants to do it badly enough . . . (Age 30, designer)
>
> . . . I am grateful that my parent let me live my life even though it may mean injury . . .(Age 29, minister)
>
> . . . My parents taught me to accept my condition as a fact but not as a handicap . . . (Age 31, writer)
>
> . . . After my service experience I found I had to stay away from "momma" (respectfully). After getting married we located approximately . . . miles from where everyone knew of my troubles. Present neighbors and friends regard my trouble considerably different than those who knew me and "momma" as a child. (Age 34, appraiser)
>
> I am much better off since I went away to school. Because my parents were not around, I treated small hemorrhages early before they had a chance to get worse. When at home my parents would force me to go to bed and curtail my activities, so I left minor hemorrhages unattended in order to draw no attention to them, hoping they would get no worse; 50 percent did, but 50 percent became major. Away from home I could attend to minor hemorrhages and still keep active.
>
> It is very hard for anyone but the experienced sufferer himself to know what should really be done . . . (Age 26, operations research analyst)

Some respondents who had engaged in strenous activities in childhood and adolescence, or who as adults were now doing so in work or recreation, stated they had suffered few or no physical ill-effects. Others said that the resulting psychological well-being was well worth any pain or injury engendered by such actions.

> Try to make their lives as normal as possible. It's hard to always hear "no" to everything you would like to do. My parents have encouraged me to do as much as possible even when I know they must have been sick with worry. Sometimes I've landed in the hospital from something I've done but it was worth it. (Age 17, still in school)
>
> I found the more careful I was the more I got hurt. So in grade school I done just as the others done and I got along a lot better and I had less joint bleeding. (Age 22, never employed)

A frequent comment was that parents should not let the child be aware of their own fears regarding his possible injury. Also mentioned often were the damaging effects of parental blame for hemorrhaging, financial difficulties, or any parental attitudes that would provoke guilt and anxiety in the hemophilic child.

> Treat him as you would a normal child. Don't let him know that it worries you, for this will cause him to dread the bleeding spells more . . . (Age 29, shipping clerk)
>
> Briefly, to parents I feel their first duty beside the normal responsibility of parenthood is to fight the outlooks of oversheltering, financial worries due to illness caused by the child, comparisons to other handicapped afflictions. (Age 25, commercial artist)
>
> Don't be over protective. Provide the proper background for the child for employment or self-support. Don't show disappointment, discouragement or resentment because of the child's handicap or affliction. Don't discuss financial stresses in regard to medical aid for the child. Avoid giving the impression that he is different from other children. Encourage him to be independent, but sociable. (Age 31, self-employed barber)
>
> For mother and father not to fuss at child when he has an attack. Face the fact that it could not be helped, keep him in the mood that everything will be okay. Teach him the fact that he will have to stay in bed for long periods and have very few playmates and these playmates must be instructed of his condition. (Age 43, self-employed dairy owner)
>
> Do not overprotect and don't tell the child that every time he has a hemmorrage it is because he done something he should not have done. (Age 23, technician, blood bank)

The need for parental emotional support, particularly during episodes of bleeding, was often expressed.

> Have patients with them at all times, especially when they are sick, because no one know what pain it is . . . (Age 26, clerk-bookkeeper)
>
> Parents of hemophiliacs should not belittle or harangue a child for his natural desire to want to participate in physically active games . . . Extreme caution should be taken in use of pain-relieving drugs. Parents and family should remember that companionship during the time that the pain is most excruciating is as good a palliative as Demerol®, Seconal®, or what have you . . . (Age 27, teacher)

Goals, Activities

"Goals, achievement, and activities" was the second most frequent category of comment. It was related to the "normality" category, since the implied or stated purpose for the "normality" advice was to foster normal development and self-sufficiency. The expectation was that the overprotected child will be socially and economically dependent as an adult, while the child who is permitted freedom will achieve a greater degree of self-sufficiency, independence, or vocational success. This emphasis on the emerging self-sufficient adult, ready to compete on the labor market and living normally among his peers, characterizes the advice the majority of hemophiliacs would offer to parents.

> See that their child gets an education. Encourage him to take an interest in many things. Don't wait until he is back "on his fee" to start taking an interest in things. Study and play with him, so that when he does grow up he'll have an idea of what he can do. Hemorrhaging causes a lot of damage through the years and if he can learn when he is younger he'll be better fitted to make his way through life. I thought that when I got through school life would be easier. It is far from that because you've got to do things on your own, and make your own way. It is "easier" when he is younger. His parents are there in time of need. But when he grows up they won't always be there, and like any boy—in his heart he'll want to make his own way. So start now to see that he is educated for the future. (Age 25, glass-blower)

> . . . don't be quite so apprehensive about a hemophiliac child and/or adult, after all, they are not at all as fragile as most parents think. Develop his vocational interest and guide him into something he can do physically, but don't neglect his general education. As he grows into adulthood, let him be his own individual self, in other words, don't keep telling him what he can and can't do. Let him make his own decisions, this is the only way he can grow up, so to speak, hemophilia or not. (Age 27, never employed)

> I would say for them to get all the schooling they could get because it is tough without it. (Age 32, gauge repairman)

> See that they go to school and get Educated. there's nothing like having a shop or your on business . . . I have been lucky so far as workking and helping a family. If I had my on shop I wouldn't have to worry about people or bosses knowing of my condition. There's nothing like a good Education. (Age 36, truck driver)

Some respondents stressed the idea that emphasis should be placed on intellectual development as a compensation for necessary physical restrictions.

> . . . give them the best possible education in a line of work that can

be performed with little physical effort—as art—some musical instruments—mathematics or science and engineering. We have to realize we cannot compete physically so we must excell mentally or have a talent to earn our way. (Age 40, optical technician)

Emotional Adjustment

Closely related to the advice stressing goals and independence or self-sufficiency was concern for the emotional adjustment of the hemophiliac. Some respondents felt that frequent onsets of illness and pain, with the resulting confinement and frustration, would be psychologically damaging to the child. Psychiatric consultation or care was often recommended.

Many respondents felt that the overprotected child will become emotionally, as well as physically, handicapped, while children who are encouraged toward normal childhood activities, preparation for future goals, and the development of self-reliance will be better adjusted and better able to cope with the special problems of hemophilia.

> My recommendation is an emphasis on intellectual development, either professional, or vocational education in a field within the child's limitations. The child will be a better adjusted individual if he is given as much freedom as possible in learning what his physical limitations are. The child should be treated like a normal child to the greatest extent possible. (Age 21, still in school)

> Do not "pamper" him more than his brothers and sisters, as it will complicate his future relations with all people he may meet. Teach him to be interested in mental work—tone down the physical activity to his particular ability to handle it. He must learn to like people and not feel sorry for himself. (Age 42, watch repair)

> A hemophiliac must not be left to draw up in a shell. He should lead as much of a normal life as possible. At the earliest time his condition should be makde known to him so he would understand why there are certain activities he cannot join in. Above all he should lead a fairly normal, happy life with his friends and family. (Age 27, spray painter)

> On this subject I have strong feelings. The main thing is for the parents to treat the child as a *normal person* as much as possible. Don't treat them as a boy that is "different." Watch them, but *don't let the child become aware of the extra care.* This is difficult, but my *parents were successful.* (Age 22, teacher)

Adjust to the reality of life not to hemophilia. A not well-adjusted hemophiliac is unable to take care of himself. But it isn't easy and he needs help. I had help. (Age 39, director of public relations)

Teach them early in life what they can and cannot do, and stress those things they can do and prepare them as best you can to do those things.

Don't continually tell the child that they may out-grow H and give them a false hope.

My mother made the mistake of forever telling me that I would never be able to do anything and I believed her. (Age 34, unemployed; part-time insurance agent)

Medical Advice

Comments on medical advice stressed three main areas: obtaining good medical care, care of the teeth, and specific recommendations for physical regimen and diet. Treatment recommendations included the use of cold packs, bandages, vitamins, transfusions and plasma. Many stressed the importance of finding a good doctor who is familiar with hemophilia and remaining under his care.

Concern for the care of teeth and mention of dental problems were common. From our study it appears that dental problems are a major factor for many hemophiliacs, regardless of the severity of the case. One of the problems, aside from the feasibility of dental care according to the individual case, is finding dentists who have the special skill or willingness to work with hemophiliacs. Some hemophiliacs with no other major problems related to their disease said their teeth are a constant source of discomfort and pain, affecting other areas of their lives. From a medical standpoint, it is important to develop better techniques of dental care for hemophiliacs and a larger group of dentists specially trained to provide such care.

Restrictions

A few respondents stressed restrictions or watchful care.

. . . teach their children to be careful of injuring or cutting their selves or engaging in rough play. Or dangerous sports. (Age 60, farmer)

> . . . stress the fact that the child must be very very careful while he is a pre-teener and a teenager, because his condition will improve with age, mine did, but I was already crippled by then. (Age 32, never employed)

> It's not too good for them to run much and play ball, and swimming and to be wrestle and to keep sharp knives and other sharp instruments away from them. (Age 22, never employed)

But such comments were rare. Many who advised restrictions showed concern as well for the interrelated emotional involvement and for the development of goal striving behavior.

> . . . try to keep the child away from partisipation in sports such as football and baseball.
>
> The main thing is to not let the young child do various strenuous activities, but do not shelter him. Both of which could hinder him in later life, particularly the latter. (Age 22, still in school)

> Provide as early as possible realization of limitations, attendance at regular school; the patient must realize early that there is no cure and that avoidance of stressful play will prolong onset of permanent joint involvement. Parent should avoid psychological involvement through expert guidance. (Age 46, university professor)

> Restrict his physical activities if severity warrants it. Do not make him feel he is different than other children. Encourage him to get as much education as possible. Teach him how to protect himself from injury and how to care for injuries. Treat him as a normal child. (Age 26, clerk)

> Teach them to know their physical limitations—brains and thinking will have to become topes. Do not baby or become overly protective. A some what normal life minus sports can be lived. Stay away from all harmful or stimulating food and drinking and smoking. Life a clean life. (Age 41, radio mechanic)

While a number of examples of this kind of advice are provided, it should be recalled that only 15 percent of the entire sample recommended restricting the child.

Other Advice

Advice concerning having children and on drug addiction are important, not because of their frequency of occurrence in the responses but because of their possible significance to the hemophilic population.

Very few respondents mentioned problems resulting from the use of drugs, yet the danger of drug addiction for the hemophilic population has been generally recognized by doctors, and many hemophiliacs seem aware of this danger. Fifteen respondents mentioned problems or possible problems associated with the use of pain-killing drugs, either advising parents to avoid them, or stating that they themselves at one time were addicted, or that they were aware that this was a problem for other hemophiliacs.

Five respondents advised parents of hemophilic children to avoid further childbearing, and two said, "Put them to sleep." Eighteen hemophiliacs felt that hemophiliacs themselves should not father children. Respondents who gave such advice often expressed dissatisfaction with their own situation, their lack of success in vocational achievement, or felt they had suffered greatly in connection with their disease, as in the following example:

> It is a very expensive disease. It costs us over $1000 a year for plasma & medicine. My wife is an R.N. and gives me plasma at home and so I have not had to go to the hospital lately. Before this I went to a clinic in S.F. but there you do what their Drs. say even if they want to experiment such as surgery. I could not even have my own business without leaving someone fill in when I am suddenly bedridden with a hemorrhage. I feel carriers should adopt children rather than risk having a hemophiliac. (Age 37, self employed)

Since most married hemophiliacs tend to have children however, and in view of the scarcity of such advice, it seems likely that only a few hemophiliacs feel they should not have children.

Other advice which occurred frequently was the need for clinical understanding of the disease on the part of the parents and of the child. Parents were advised by many respondents to seek consultation from physicians and through the hemophilia associations to learn all they could about the disease and to inform their children of the facts of hemophilia so that they might understand the problems they encounter, the need for care and restrictions, and learn to care for themselves.

Some respondents emphasized the advisability of "playing down" or disguising the hemophiliac's condition so that a normal life pattern could be followed, to avoid social stigma or isolation, or for other reasons. On the other hand, some respondents advised openness with regard to the child's condition in order to establish a realistic life pattern for social protection, or because "there's nothing to be ashamed of."

EMPLOYMENT

The most frequent negative remarks dealt with employers' attitudes toward hiring and/or keeping hemophiliacs, or the lack of opportunities for advancement because of such attitudes.

> The most serious problem I have had is finding work even in fields that I know because of hemophilia. An educational program beamed at employers explaining that hemophiliacs are more conscientious than the average person and is less apt to leave a job once he is hired. (Age 39, manufacturing engineer)
>
> I feel that hemophilia is a drawback as far as my trade is concerned as many businessmen do not understand and are afraid of the word. And will limit my chances of reaching my goal . . . (Age 34, glass blower)
>
> I have went for a job menny times, and they turn me down when they see i have a Brase on, So they begain asking questions why i have it on. I wants to work to help my mother with the other children. but i be turn down all the time . . . (Age 18, still in school)
>
> I don't envy the younger fellows who are coming of working age, because it gets very discouraging when you have the ability or education, and yet be turned down because of health conditions . . . (Age 27, insurance sales)
>
> For myself I am not asking any special favors. Although on my job where I work my record proves me to be excellent in some duties and competent in all duties, but I cannot get my steps or salary and raises because I have this Hemophiliac condition. May I ask can anything be done about this. I am only asking what is righfully mine and not for special favors. (Age 51, cook)
>
> When my Hemophilia was diagnosed my employer lowered me to a Janitor Job and kept me there 5 years. I was finally able to convince company doctor to give me a release for general work. He says it is on my Responsibility. However at my age I couldn't see being a Janitor for the rest of my life regardless of consequences. I work for a large corporation . . . employing thousands of men. They could easily find suitable jobs for Handicapped Workers. Instead they just do not want to be bothered. They employ thousands of able bodied office workers. I am presently laid off. (Age 34, manual labor–steel)

These comments show that hemophiliacs perceive employer attitudes as one of the most important barriers to vocational achievement. They stress two important ideas: that employers' negative attitudes are due to lack of information about hemophilia and the hemophiliacs' actual abilities and potential; and, that hemophiliacs can accomplish more than the general public—employers included—gives them credit for. Fewer of the respondents blamed their hemophilia per se for their dissatisfaction with their vocational achievement, but rather tended to blame society, especially employers. Insurance companies and medical departments of companies were blamed also.

Not all comments about employers were negative, however. The following quotations show that some respondents have found good work situations.

> Due to my employers understanding I have been able to keep my job. The help of the other employees when I am having hemorrhages enable me to keep up with the work. Because of the type of work I am in there is no schedule to meet and you do the work as it comes in. Thus far I have been very lucky in my employment situation.(Age 27, material expediter)

> A hemophiliac has many problems that he has to contend with. When I am working I try to work extra hard, so when I am sick it will be taken into consideration. I have found that most employers will work with you. But you have to remember that there is still a job to be done and you can't blame an employer for being concerned when you are out sick a lot. (Age 25, proofreader)

> Whenever I have missed working I have always endeavored to work overtime in order to compensate for loss of time due to my affliction.
>
> The employers I have worked for, especially the most recent one, have been most considerate.
>
> Some employers are not truthfull as to whether they are considerate toward a hemophiliacs condition. They hesitate to tell you directly. (Age 51, engineer)

> My work is very hard but I like it. And my boss is very nice to me. Like I had some dental work done and had a very bad hemorrage from it. I was in the hospital 7 days and the first night twenty of my friends came to give me blood.
>
> So after all I think I am very fortinate to have good friends. (Age 25, sheet metal worker)

Such remarks are encouraging and offer a hopeful direction for counseling and for other aspects of vocational rehabilitation. They show that there are sympathetic employers who are willing to accept some of the limitations associated with hemophilia and that there are types of work situations where the limitations are minimally felt, particularly absenteeism. Such employers and forms of work should be located, in order to expand the potential work environments available to the hemophiliac. Most hemophiliacs are probably unaware of existing possibilities since they have few means to discover them. Counselors and vocational rehabilitation workers should be able to provide this information, but must first obtain it themselves.

The comments further reveal a need for employer education regarding the actual potential of hemophiliacs. A glance at the job titles listed at the ends of the quotations gives an indication of the range of employment of which these respondents are capable, if given the opportunity.

Employment—Further Descriptive Comments

The following comments additionally exemplify positive vocational situations:

> . . . I have been in the retail shoe Business (for myself) since I was 19 years old (1923) and nobody has worked or does work any Harder than I do. I am not nor ever was crippled or Handicapped in any manner. My employees who are much younger and Have no affliction cannot keep up with me as far as work, effort and ambition is concerned.
>
> My main difficulty through the years Have Been occasional Bleeding of the gums and being confined to a Hospital for approximate 2 weeks after an extraction. (Age 57, self-employed, store)

> With the help of my parents Voc Rehab. & Drs. I have my own barber shop doing ok. am married and have two husky boys. A Good Helper in my Wife. I have a two chair shop in a county seat town. Have a good biss. (Age 22, self-employed barber)

> . . . I am working at a job that is ideal for a hemophiliac. In my Department my two co-workers also have handicaps. So that when

one is out sick the other two carry the burden of three. But a situation such as this is very rare. I have been working since I was 16 years old. I have gone from job to job till I found this one. At which I have been working for 8 years. The main concern of Hemophiliacs is not finding a job but keeping one. And if he has responsibility what to do for money when he is not working . . . If some sort of financing aid can be given to him at these times much will have been done to improve his lot. (Age 38, clerk)

. . . Scholastic and professional opportunities have usually opened for me at times when I've been ready for them. I originally planned to be a science writer, but became fascinated with math and did well in it. I am a second rate mathematician, but am inventive enough to find my work thoroughly satisfying. My salary is about $9,200–medical bills still loom large, but a new insurance plan is helping. I hope other hemophiliacs will consider applied mathematics as a career–it's a growing field. I feel that my relative success is due to (1) learning to love to read, omnivorously as a child; (2) some fortunate contact with good teachers at the right times; (2) very patient bosses; (4) very patient wife and family. (Age 28, mathematician)

The following comments describe a variety of situations and are useful in that they provide a broader picture of existing vocational situations in which hemophiliacs are engaged.

. . . When I was young I was told by my parents that I would never be able to work. When I graduated from high school I was determined to prove to them that they were wrong. I went job hunting two days after graduation and found a job on a farm. I didn't tell them of my condition. I drove a tractor, fed and helped care for about 200 aberdiene Angus cattle. I like the out-door work and my employer kept me until cold weather set in and work was slow.

I have been working at various jobs ever since. I never told my employers of my condition for fear of not getting the job. So at most jobs when I began losing time I got laid off. I'm presently employed with . . . and have been for 3 years. They know of my condition and give me jobs that are not dangerous to my health. I hope I can stay there indefinitly but live in constant fear of loseing it . . . (Age 38, plastic molding)

. . . Up to this time most of my jobs have been part time, either in the summer or at Christmas time . . . Some of them are: mail carrier, type-setter, paper boy, cutting grass, and other similar, normal occupations. (Age 20, still in school)

Ranched at home with father and brother. Too strenuous. Took watch repair for 18 mo. Worked 65 days to gain shop experience. Am now converting large house to 3 rental apts. and own shop and apartments. Do some watch work also, but primarily engaged in carpentry etc. to get house rented. Am on last apt. Will complete soon and open Repair shop on full scale. Hope to have partial living from 6 hrs. work daily, rest from rentals. Should be OK (Age 44, watch repair)

I am now serving in the United States Navy enlisted in 1958 am serving a four year term have not had any trouble with being hemophilian. I have told them when I enlisted. I am aboard a minesweeper and am a Yoeman 3rd class . . . (Age 22, sailor)

Problems of Hemophilia in Relation to Employment

Chapter 6 gave details of the actual situation of hemophiliacs in relation to their work. The following comments illustrate the respondents' *feelings and perceptions* of their work situations, when problems were experienced. Absenteeism is a major concern, and closely related are feelings of insecurity because of the unpredictability of the hemophiliac's state of health. The feeling of "not knowing from one day to the next" was often expressed.

The unemployed and the never-employed tended to emphasize the disabling or interfering effects of hemophilia, particularly with regard to absenteeism and unpredictability of tenure. If their comments were about employment, the employed more frequently blamed employers and lack of education and complained of low wages. Thus, the comments suggest that the successful tended to blame or criticize society for any felt failure or dissatisfaction, while the unsuccessful more often blamed their hemophilia.

I work according to my condition and pain which I might have, as I never know when this condition will arise . . . (Age 44, unemployed)

The kind of jobs open to a hemophiliac are to few, and even the ones that a hemophiliac can do, the uncertainty of his condition holds him back from trying. Self confidence in most hemophiliacs is very bad and he will not exert himself to attain any kind of success . . . (Age 29, never employed)

I am well satisfied with the job I have now, only I'm afraid I'm going to lose it because I already have lost time. I worked 7 days and lost 5 worked 6 days and at present I am off because a severe pain in my knee joint which developed as I was sleeping last night. Even though I have a government job with social security, which hire the handicapped. I was told that they couldn't tolerate chronic absenteeism.

If I lose this job the same thing will happen on future jobs. If I'm lucky to get anything else. (Age 20, file clerk)

If it were not for my elbos I would louse very little time from work. they are swollen, stiff and very painful most of the time. I don't think there is anything that can be done about it. Besides I can not take time out from work because of money and I would louse my job because of the time it would take to take care of them.

When you are like me, you do anything to get or keep a job. If you are in pain, it takes money to stop it and if you don't work you don't eat and so on . . . (Age 30, lathe operator)

I wroke full time but is very difficult some time I barely limp around the pain in ankle. Havent found any reliefe as yet. (Age 32, unemployed carpenter)

. . . 1. Even though I've worked in my present job for 10 years and never been fired, with little chance that I will be now. The wages are low and with time lost even lower.

2. I am afread to look for another better paying job because of the time I have to be out and the lack of a better education.

3. Increasing arthritic pains in my legs, sometimes I can hardly walk. And a constant fatigued feeling. (Age 32, file clerk)

I feel I could do more and work better in some other position. My current job does not allow for my promotion or advancement. I work part time as a free lance photographer to help finance my medical expenses. My present financial situation is limited.

The most serious problem in getting enough blood donors finding other employment with the education I have. (Age 37, clerk)

1. Insurance . . . so vital in the positions I am qualified.

2. Financial backing–Each time I get ahead a little bit I get sick and use all my reserve.

3. Improper Schooling–The technical knowledge I was born with more than enough–but it is the basic lack of English and spelling that is very important in my line of work . . .

4. If I were healthy, it wouldn't be so important, because I know mechanics inside out–precision and heavy mechanics–I have worked in garages on cars since I was big enough to reach the accelerator on a car, but now I'm older, it is just too hard on my physically.

5. People just do not understand hemophilia (Age 28, instr. tech.)

EDUCATION

About 11 percent of the respondents, mostly in the still-in-school group, discussed education in their comments, although a larger percentage mentioned the need for a good education in their advice to parents. The remarks could be classified as positive or negative, having to do with how the respondent evaluated his own school experiences. The positive remarks dealt with school achievement or pride in accomplishment. Absenteeism was mentioned as a problem by 31 percent of the still in school, and 15 percent indicated they were unsuccessful in school, were discouraged, or otherwise had problems in school. However, 58 percent indicated they were pleased with their experiences or doing well in school.

The never-employed and the unemployed tended to comment that they had not received sufficient education, that they were unable to attend or complete school, or that absenteeism had been a major problem.

The employed, on the other hand, tended to say they were successful in school (44%); however, 28 percent said they felt handicapped by insufficient education, 8 percent said absenteeism had been a problem, and 6 percent said they had been unable to attend school.

Where criticisms of school systems or individual schools were offered, the idea was stressed that the inflexibility of school policies hampered the young hemophiliac in participating at the expected grade level for his age. Since absenteeism is the major problem in relation to obtaining education, it is often necessary for the hemophiliac to make up school work, take tests at later dates, and have tutoring. From the comments offered by the respondents, it appears that most hemophiliacs feel that education at a regular school is the best situation for normal development. Yet, because of absenteeism they have difficulty in keeping up with their classmates and some respondents stated that they had been held back in school because they had fallen behind in their work or had missed too many examinations. They felt that the schools should be more flexible in allowing them to make up missed work or examinations.

From other data previously reported, it appears that such retardation leads to school drop-out before completion or even entrance into high school. Some of the still in school commented that they were behind in grade level for their age and *there is some evidence that hemophiliacs tend to be at least one and a half to two years behind in grade level.* The extremely high relationship found between school success and vocational and personal adjustment indicates that this is an important area for future study.

Several respondents said they had been refused admission to schools and universities on the basis of high risk. Some mentioned experiences which indicated a lack of understanding on the part of school personnel of the need for personal development of the hemophiliac and of his special problems. A few mentioned they had been made to feel the focus of attention by their teachers, and a few said their teachers had felt that as students they had no future, discouraging scholastic achievement. It seems apparent that many school personnel would benefit from education which could provide understanding of hemophilia and of the developmental needs and potentialities of the hemophiliac child.

Many hemophiliacs, however, stated that they were successful in school—although often their accomplishment, because of absenteeism, had taken them longer than the average nonhemophiliac. Some credited the extra help they had received from teachers for the fact that they were able to complete their schooling. Several mentioned that they were attending a university, working toward advanced degrees; others were preparing to do so; some were carrying full graduate-study loads and working halftime as teaching and research assistants. The range of educational achievement for the respondents was wide, and it appears that environmental factors could often account for success or nonsuccess in addition to hemophilia-related factors. Parental encouragement and the functioning of individual school systems, including the availability of tutors and special programs or policies with regard to the hemophiliac, appear to be two important factors.

RELATIONSHIP TO SOCIETY, SOCIAL EXPERIENCE

Social Barriers to Success and Adjustment

Not all hemophiliacs feel they have problems associated either with society or with hemophilia. Some respondents, in fact, stated they had none, but the majority probably are concerned to some degree with the following problems.

Lack of Public Information and Understanding

The overriding social problem might be expressed in the following manner: "The public is too uninformed about hemophilia" or "most people just do not understand the hemophiliac, what he is capable of . . . " Lack of information and of understanding by the public are perceived by many hemophiliacs as the bases for employer discrimination along with lack of training or educational opportunities and opportunity for job advancement. Such lack of information and understanding is considered the source of emphasis on the disabilities of hemophiliacs rather than on their capabilities and potential. The emphasis on disability results in loss of opportunity, and occasionally in social isolation and personal discouragement. For this reason public ignorance often underlies concealment of hemophilia. Some hemophiliacs relocate their residences, in order to avoid social stigma and discrimination, in an environment where no one knows of their condition.

> We want to be treated as normal people not as a baby . . . Job opportunities are our biggest problem we face as things stand now. We are limited as far as insurance companies are concerned even the accident industrial board in the state puts such a restriction on us we don't stand a chance of a job we want. People don't realize we know what we can do and cannot do. We are more cautious than the regular worker but still people are not informed enough about hemophilia. They just know that we are bleeders and that we have a lot of trouble stopping a cut . . . (Age 21, machinist)

> My greatest handicap was to over come the fact of people having pity in a small town and constantly talking of bleeding. I am living a new life, have an excellent position after working hard for a college

education, but would never have had this job if anyone knew I was a hemophiliac. (Age 26, sales rep.)

. . . the main problem with any hemophiliac is pride. He does not want to admit that he has any limitations. This in turn causes a degree of carelessness. If the normal side of the average hemophiliac were made known to the public, the problem would be less. My grade school classmates always laughed because teachers told them I was fragile. This was dispised, hence I was out to prove my life was as normal as theirs by doing things I shouldn't have. This is the source of any complication I have today. (Age 23, engineer)

. . . As I said, the only real disappointment was the refusal of a university to accept me on the grounds that my hemophilia would put too much responsibility on the school . . . I, as a hemophiliac, have made my adjustments and try to lead as normal and full life as is possible. It is the people who will not let us lead our lives the way that we see fit that are our main obstacles. (Age 21, univ. student–works part time)

. . . Most employers are reluctant to run the risk of employing a hemophiliac. Most people (M.D.'s included) know little about hemophilia, in fact are misinformed–they do not realize there are variations from individual to individual–press releases are execrable and articles such as the recent Post article are damnable. I feel very strongly that they do more harm than good. These articles are particularly harmful to adult hemophiliacs who have arrived at some stability in their condition. With the more widespread use of plasma more hemophiliacs are living to adulthood, and there is a need to emphasize the difference between an adult and a child hemophiliac–certainly the public isn't being informed of this fact. The fear of hemophilia and hemophiliacs can have serious consequences. I've had doctors refuse to treat me, as well as employers refuse to hire me. There was some question as to whether I could obtain a Teachers' Certificate because of this . . .

I had some difficulty in obtaining a graduate award but fortunately my advisor and 2 or 3 other members of the dept. here, took the time and trouble to find out more about hemophilia and how it affects me . . .

I feel that one of the most tragic mistakes my parents made was to let it be generally known that I had this condition. Fortunately we moved half-way across the continent before I entered high school and I was able to start over with only a few people knowing about my hemophilia and I was able to have a much more normal life. At present probably 5% of my friends, acquaintances, and associates know I have hemophilia, and it is never discussed or used–the limitations that I must impose on myself are accepted as a matter of course . . . (Age 31, univ. grad. student–Research Asst.)

While the lack of public understanding was emphasized mainly with relation to employer discrimination, the above examples illustrate other negative effects frequently mentioned by the respondents. Peer group and other social contacts, state agencies, insurance companies, physicians, welfare agencies, educators, parents, and the press are often described as poorly informed and as providing barriers to the hemophiliac in one form or another. Additionally, some respondents felt that the lack of public information and interest had an adverse effect on the amount of research conducted on hemophilia and on the hemophiliac's financial situation, including the problems associated with blood replacement. *The hemophiliac, then, often feels there is a wide gulf between him and the rest of society as a result of disinterest and misinformation.* He often feels stigmatized by attitudes of pity and of fear and feels that such attitudes have practical effects in loss of opportunity and benefits which might otherwise be afforded him.

Groups and Organizations Discussed by the Respondents

The Field of Medicine

About 10 percent of the 720 respondents who provided written comments expressed criticism of their medical care. The most frequent criticism was lack of knowledge on the part of doctors regarding the medical aspects, diagnosis, and treatment of hemophilia. According to these respondents, they have encountered doctors who were unfamiliar with or barely acquainted with hemophilia. Some doctors have been skeptical of the respondents' diagnoses and have recommended and provided ill-advised treatment such as major surgery, withheld blood transfusions, refused patient's deferment from the armed forces, refused treatment for, or mistreated pain, caused unnecessary pain, and left severe internal bleeding untreated due to faulty diagnosis and "neglect."

Such experiences have apparently been frequently

encountered by hemophiliacs and probably supply the basis for such respondents' comments as "stay away from quack doctors" and "find a good M.D., hematologist, or hemophilia specialist, and stick with him." About 5 percent of the seven hundred respondents said they had received good treatment, credited their doctor or a particular medical staff with excellent care and rehabilitative treatment. Those who spoke positively of the medical profession usually pointed to a specific doctor or care center, while those who spoke negatively usually applied their remarks to the profession in general. Some who felt they had received poor medical care were grateful to have finally found a "good" doctor under whose care they planned to remain.

Hemophiliacs often feel that by the time they reach adulthood they know more about their physical condition and requirements than do many medical personnel, particularly those in the lower echelons of hospital staffs. Some respondents complained of mistreatment in hospitals and that nurses and nurses aides "would not listen," although as patients they often knew what treatment they should and should not have.

Other complaints concerning physicians included their disinterest or lack of understanding of the psychological effects of physical trauma, and enforced immobilization on hemophiliac children, and refusal to give preventive transfusions when the patient felt he needed them. Several respondents said they and other hemophiliacs of their acquaintance had been "experimented on" ill-advisedly. Medical departments of large companies were blamed for job refusal.

From the positive remarks regarding doctors, it appears that superior medical care is available to hemophiliacs, but sometimes the individual hemophiliac cannot locate the proper physician or hospital facility. It appears, too, that many physicians who treat hemophiliacs are insufficiently knowledgeable about it, while respondents who live in outlying or rural areas are restricted in their choice of doctor, although some of them had found family doctors who are highly skilled and competent in their care. By and large, the respondents who received care from the principal hemophilia centers indicated satisfaction with and gratitude toward their doctors.

Public Assistance, Vocational Rehabilitation and Social Security

Only fourteen respondents said they were receiving Social Security or disability payments. The Vocational Rehabilitation Administration had provided 12 percent of the respondents with rehabilitative care in some form, such as counseling or job training, and a small percentage of the respondents indicated they had at some time received financial aid from public or private welfare agencies.

Yet, according to the written remarks, financial problems are uppermost in importance for a large portion of the respondents. Hospital and doctor's bills, blood replacement, and other medical costs were frequently mentioned. The written remarks indicate that, despite their need, hemophiliacs receive very little outside financial assistance. Some respondents said the VRA has provided or was expected to provide assistance in their job training or placement. Others said they had been refused help by VRA or had been offered aid which was impractical for them or that VRA was able to offer training but could not help in finding jobs. Some respondents indicated they were unaware of the existence of VRA, stating they wished there were an agency which could help to train hemophiliacs and to find jobs for them.

Suggestions for financial relief were offered, e.g. reduced income tax, greater availability of insurance coverage, public fund-raising, early pensions. Indications are that most hemophiliacs do not desire to live on welfare, but some feel that special assistance should be provided in times of greatest financial need. It appears, too, that some hemophiliacs do not know where to look for financial and other rehabilitative assistance, and some have been refused assistance by various agencies. According to the respondents, some of the reasons for refusal by the agencies were financial ineligibility, too great a degree of handicap, work not available, and discontinuance of financial assistance for education because of frequent absence from school. Some of the reports indicate that welfare and rehabilitation agencies are not sufficiently informed regarding the special problems and potential abilities of hemophiliacs and that their policies with regard to hemophiliacs are only vaguely formulated. This conclusion is tentatively drawn since it is based mainly on the self-reports of the involved clients, yet the problem is of sufficient magnitude that it bears further study, as exemplified in the following comment:

> . . . I would like to attend college this fall but due to my illness and the great expense that goes with it my family can't afford to send me. I asked the Rehabilitation to help send me 2 yrs. ago but the man I talked to didn't understand my condition and seemed to think I could make it on my own. So many people have never heard of hemophilia and its hard for them to understand why a blood disease can prevent you from working and especially if you look as healthy as I do . . .,(Age 21, roofer's helper employed by father)

PHYSICAL ASPECTS

About 50 percent of the eighty-two respondents who mentioned causes of hemorrhaging said that physical activity, whether strenuous or not, had little or nothing to do with onset of hemorrhaging. Twenty-five respondents said that rough play as a child or strenuous work had led to hemorrhaging or crippling. The remainder offered various opinions on causes of hemorrhages which included weather conditions, poor general physical condition, and diet.

Over 140 respondents described severe afflictions resulting from their hemophilia, including paralysis, lung collapse, hepatitis, impaired eyesight, amputations, kidney damage, dental problems, arthritis and other joint problems, and some severe non–hemophilia-related conditions which cannot be corrected by surgery because of hemophilia.

Severe, almost continuous pain was described by fifty-three respondents, in addition to many who mentioned the effects of pain on the hemophilic child in their advice to parents.

SELF-VIEW, COPING MECHANISMS, ATTITUDES TOWARD HEMOPHILIA

A total of 377 respondents provided statements descriptive of their attitudes toward hemophilia or illustrative ways of coping with this pervasive life situation. The ways in which the respondent viewed his functioning, his perceived potentialities as a hemophiliac, expressions of the ways in which hemophilia was seen to determine or to have an effect on the general life situations of hemophiliacs were interpreted as reflecting attitudes toward the respondent's own life situations as a hemophiliac. Such attitudes appear to bear a strong relationship to the effective functioning of the indivdual. While the remarks themselves may be representative of the hemophilic population, the distribution of the remarks may not be, since not all of the respondents referred to this area of concern. Those who commented in this area tended to give positive answers. On a continuum from positive to negative, with the general tone inferred from all the comments, 66 percent of all the 720 written comments were classified as positive, while 28 percent were classified as negative. With regard to the attitudinal remarks made by 377 respondents, the greatest percentage were of a positive nature.

The remarks were classified in two additional ways: those which seemed to express attitudes toward hemophilia, along with adaptation or coping mechanisms; and remarks which seemed to express how the respondent was functioning, his view of himself and his life situation in relation to hemophilia. There were 519 comments made by the 377 respondents; these comments were coded into these two categories, representing an overlap of 142 comments.

View of Self

A total of 303 remarks were coded into the following nine categories:

1. Respondent said he had *no* problems from hemophilia, lives just like anyone else. N = 14

2. Hemophilia interferes minimally with functioning, very little trouble from hemophilia, leads a normal life. N = 38

3. He is satisfied, pleased with his functioning, "I'm doing o.k.," "I'm lucky," "when I'm not sick I lead a full life." N = 87

4. Has performed better at work, socially, or in other aspects than other hemophiliacs; has more fortunate circumstances; has had less trouble than others.	N = 21
5. Is active, hard-working; has interests, goals; tries to keep up normal activities despite discomfort.	N = 40
6. Has made an extra effort in school, socially, work, because of hemophilia.	N = 15
7. Hemophilia does *not* hold him back from achieving (despite problems).	N = 13
8. Hemophilia holds him back from achieving in work, other goals, activities; feels left out of life; has many life problems from hemophilia.	N = 47
9. He can't expect to achieve, live normally; "I'm too far gone," can't work; indicated he felt hopeless, helpless, discouraged.	N = 28
	303

It can be seen that 75 percent of the remarks (categories 1-7) are in a positive direction. How representative this distribution is of the population is unknown, but the findings do indicate that a negative self-view is not necessarily typical of hemophiliacs. Despite physical and social handicaps, the main source of satisfaction appears to center around striving and activity. This self-view may differ from the views held by the public who often expect hemophiliacs to be dependent and dissatisfied in their life situations.

A total of 216 comments were classified in eight categories describing ways in which the respondents handle their situations as hemophiliacs, or expressing feelings about hemophilia as a barrier to adjustment and achievement (see Table XXXVIII).

The high severe and the intermediate-high-major groups offered complaints more frequently than did the other two groups, although 37 percent of the high severe said they minimize their condition or stressed activity rather than preoccupation with disability.

TABLE XXXVIII

SEVERITY IN RELATION TO ATTITUDES-ADAPTATION

	Severity			
Attitudes-Adaptation	*Low Severe (N = 70)** %	*Intermediate High-Major (N = 40)* %	*Intermediate High-Minor (N = 16)* %	*High Severe (N = 67)* %
Activity	14	5	6	12
Minimize-fighting spirit	34	33	44	25
Objectivity	20	10	25	15
Mild complaint and insecurity	16	20	13	30
Stresses affliction and strong complaint	16	33	13	18
	100	101	101	100

*N's are numbers in each group who commented in this area of response.

Table XXXIX a cross-tabulation between severity and self-view, shows that while more of the high-severe than low-severe hold a negative self-view, most of the high-severe responded in the "positive" categories. Their positive remarks tended to emphasize activity, striving, and effort more than did those of the low-severe, who more often said they had few or no problems with regard to hemophilia.

TABLE XXXIX

SEVERITY AND SELF-VIEW

	Severity			
Self-view	*Low Severe (N = 118)* %	*Intermediate High-Major (N = 54)* %	*Intermediate High-Minor (N = 19)* %	*High Severe (N = 72)* %
Few or no problems	28	7	5	5
Satisfied with functioning	28	24	26	29
Better than other hemophiliacs	10	7	0	7
Active, effort, hemophilia does not hinder	19	22	43	29
Hemophilia holds back, can't achieve	15	39	26	31
	100	99	100	101

Tables XL and XLI show that while some of the employed stressed the disabling effect of hemophilia and were dissatisfied with their accomplishment, way of life, et cetera, most gave "positive" responses. Clearly contrasted were the unemployed-never-employed, most of whom said they were dissatisfied and discouraged and who appeared to feel that hemophilia was a problem of such great magnitude that they were unable to strive, to achieve, or to live in a manner which would de-emphasize the disabling physical effects of their condition.

TABLE XL

EMPLOYMENT STATUS AND ATTITUDES-ADAPTATION

	Employment Status		
	*Employed (N = 130)**	*Still in School (N = 47)*	*Never-Employed Unemployed (N = 34)*
Attitudes-Adaptation	%	%	%
Activity	11	13	9
Minimize-fighting spirit	31	43	12
Objectivity	18	21	9
Mild complaint and insecurity	18	17	44
Stresses affliction and strong complaint	22	6	26
	100	100	100

*N's are numbers in each group who commented in this area of response.

TABLE XLI

EMPLOYMENT STATUS AND SELF-VIEW

	Employment Status		
	*Employed (N = 180)**	*Still in School (N = 79)*	*Unemployed Never-Employed (N = 44)*
Self-view	%	%	%
Few or no problems	20	15	9
Satisfied with functioning	30	38	7
Better than other hemophiliacs	8	6	2
Active, effort, hemophilia does *not* hinder	23	27	14
Hemophilia holds back, can't achieve	19	14	68
	100	100	100

*N's are number in each group who commented in this area of response.

SUMMARY

From all these data, it seems likely that the way in which the hemophiliac views his situation is strongly related to the effectiveness of his functioning in daily life, including his employment status, social adjustment, and activity level. The more emphasis he places on his disability, irrespective of the degree of severity, the less likely he is to have found an effective mode of coping or adjustment in other areas of life. While this observation is an expected one (and one which may be made concerning other forms of disability), it serves to point up an important area for action and further study.

Chapter 12

CONCLUSIONS: HEMOPHILIA—THE HOPE AND REALITY

WE have taken a wide-screen look at some key aspects of the lives of hemophiliacs, and it is now time to review and sum up our findings.

A leitmotif of this work is the belief that, broadly considered, the problems of hemophiliacs are very similar to those of other persons with a chronic physical handicap or disorder. They are problems of social understanding and acceptance, social provision and care, of the individual's being able to find a social niche that is personally rewarding and fulfilling. When they do not achieve this, hemophiliacs and others physically handicapped share some characteristics with other minority groups against whom society discriminates or excludes altogether. As the writer stated in a recent professional paper:

> These groups exhibit a *deprivation* of some material and social-psychological kind, which results in their partial exclusion and alienation from the "mainstream" of the broader society . . . [The] deprivation may be physical at base, emotional, cultural, social, educational, experiential, etc. The physically handicapped start with a physical anomaly or deprivation, but often experience a whole series of psychosocial deprivations that are a response to, a consequence of, and later a conditioning factor in negative-anticipated environmental responses.
>
> Speaking very generally, no matter what the source or origin of their deprivation, the deprived in our society have a hard row to hoe. With all its masterful technological achievements, this society does not have too much tolerance for the deviant, nor does it provide many supporting social groups for their nurturance. Individualistic and isolating tendencies, derived from the socioeconomic environment, pervade social life and individual behavior. The social norms of the society are those of individual achievement in a competitive milieu. Those who, because of a deprivation, do not have the wherewithal to compete without assistance become marked as

> deviates, sometimes as failures, and frequently their style of life both perpetuates and symbolizes the failure. Social stigma becomes attached to the deprived; it adds to their burdens, raises higher the walls over which they must climb, and by a well-studied process often becomes internalized into a negative self-image. Failure—without outside aid—becomes chronic and cyclical(12).

These broad ideas certainly apply to the situation of many hemophiliacs, but it is remarkable how many hemophiliacs have made their way, despite the social obstacles. Indeed, the primary finding of our own detailed study, one which underlies and supports most of the conclusions of this book, is this: *Hemophiliacs are capable of and often do fulfill adequate social roles in a manner and to a degree similar to that expected for the nonhemophilic population.*

Thus, the majority of the hemophiliacs we studied were found to be either employed or still-in-school; married and the head of a household which often included children; and leading active lives, both physically, and socially. Occupations were not restricted to those requiring a minimum of physical activity, but ranged from the physically sedentary to the extremely active and even hazardous. Many hemophiliacs were found to hold jobs requiring high degrees of skill, responsibility, training, and education. The income level for the employed respondents was found to be similar to that for the employed United States male working population. About 50 percent of those who were still in school were employed part time. Leisure-time activities often involved strenuous physical activity and did not necessarily lead to bleeding episodes, according to respondents' self-reports.

These findings provided a different picture of hemophiliacs from those most widely held, the popular view of hemophiliacs being that they stand in constant danger of losing life through hemorrhaging, are socially withdrawn, vocationally limited, and physically disabled.

Our second general conclusion is this: *Hemophiliacs vary in the modes and effectiveness of their personal, social, and vocational adaptation.*

Not all of the men we studied had made a "successful" adjustment or were living in a "normal" manner with regard to social role-expectations. A relatively small percentage had never been employed; others had been unemployed for a long period of time. Many of these were unmarried and dependent on their families for financial support and tended to be inactive generally as well as vocationally.

While many in this category had a relatively high degree of physical handicap resulting from hemophilia, a substantial proportion could be termed of low or intermediate severity. A distinguishing characteristic of the "unsuccessful" was the emphasis they placed on their feelings of disability, regardless of their actual disability. The unsuccessful, including those of low severity, tended to view themselves as severely disabled. In contrast, the employed tended to minimize their disability, to emphasize personal and work goals of a "normal" character, even though some of them were of high severity.

In offering advice to parents of hemophilic children, and in their other written comments, the unsuccessful most frequently recommended restriction of the child's activities and protective parental care. The unsuccessful tended to engage in fewer leisure-time activities than the employed, and their activities were most often at the sedentary end of our activity-level scale. These findings reflect the strong emphasis placed on disability by this group.

Our third conclusion confirms the findings of other investigators: *Parental overprotection or restricting the hemophilic child from participation in normal physical activities has detrimental effects on his psychosocial development.*

Those hemophiliacs who had been restricted or discouraged from normal boyhood activities reported that they either carried over a pattern of inactivity in adult life or strove in some way to overcome the effects of such overprotection. The majority of such hemophiliacs felt that an environment of overprotection with an emphasis on disability had in some way hindered their development. On the other hand, those with parents who had encouraged their active participation in school, in setting and achieving goals, and in appropriate physical activities felt that they had achieved a satisfactory personal adjustment.

We conclude that attitudes toward the situation of being a hemophiliac, the degree of emphasis placed on disability, the view of oneself as an adequate, striving individual or as dependent and disabled, and related to the early self-concepts established by the hemophiliac, apparently arise in the early self-concepts established by the hemophiliac in the context of his early family and social experience. These early-established attitudes toward self then become strongly related to the degree of "success" achieved in adulthood, in terms of employment and "normal" personal and social activities. It is apparent that these general conclusions apply as well to the situation of other chronically handicapped persons.

PROBLEMS MOST FREQUENTLY ENCOUNTERED BY HEMOPHILIACS

Among the pervasive problems which have the most far-reaching effects for hemophiliacs are the problems of absenteeism from work and school and of financial hardship.

Unanticipated, spontaneous internal bleeding often occasions absences from school and employment for hemophiliacs, resulting in a retardation or discontinuance of schooling and in vocational deficit. Financial problems throughout the lifetime of the hemophiliac stem from several sources: limited education interferes with vocational opportunities; expected absenteeism is a major reason for employers to refuse to hire hemophiliacs and one of the most frequent reasons for job loss. The expenses of medical care and the replacement of blood to hospitals and blood banks create formidable indebtedness for some hemophiliacs; so much so that at times they may forego needed medical attention that could reduce bleeding episodes and forestall physical limitation.

In addition to the employment problems and the frequent intense pain caused by their condition, most hemophiliacs are faced with a constant search for replacement to the blood banks from which they obtain transfusions. In the recent past, it has not been unusual for a single hemorrhagic episode to require thirty units or more of transfusions to bring the hemorrhaging under control. The search for blood donors has created interpersonal problems, many hemophiliacs being reluctant to request such aid constantly from friends and acquaintances, fearing stigmatization.

While absenteeism is the major interference with achievement of educational and occupational goals, it should be recognized that *not all hemophiliacs have a high number of absences per year.* Of all our employed respondents, 40 percent reported fewer than fifteen days per year absence from work due to hemophilia; 62 percent reported fewer than thirty-one. Only 20 percent of the unemployed said they had fewer than fifteen days' absences indicating the close relationship between absenteeism and unemployment.

Some additional conclusions may be derived from the above. Hemophiliacs of low and intermediate severity are good employment risks from the point of view of absenteeism, and there is some evidence that attitudes of hemophiliacs regarding their disability are related to absentee rates. These findings suggest that absenteeism might be lowered for some hemophiliacs under optimal treatment; however, it will probably continue to be a major problem.

Other problems associated with hemorrhaging include pain, hemarthropathies, interference with ongoing activities, unpredictability of occurrence of bleeding, and awareness of the possibility of death.

These problems were mentioned many times by the respondents in our study; they are more or less consistently faced by hemophiliacs in their daily lives so that their activities and their plans must be arranged to circumvent them as far as possible.

Although many hemophiliacs complained of severe and frequent pain, they also tended to advise the avoidance of pain-relieving drugs. The frequent use of such drugs has, in the past, led to a considerable, but unknown, incidence of drug-addiction among hemophiliacs. Our data did not include findings on this subject; however, we conjecture that the incidence of drug-addiction among hemophiliacs has decreased as the medical profession and hemophiliacs themselves have become aware of the danger.

From all indications, hemophiliacs consistently seek out information regarding their disease and methods of treating it. Many have placed themselves on regimens of diet or exercise under the guidance of a physician, or derived from personal experience or theories regarding their condition. Most hemophiliacs feel that, next to their own physician, they are best informed about their condition and needs. Some feel that from previous experience they are at times able to predict and even prevent hemorrhages. Management of pain is often undertaken by the hemophiliac himself, using techniques which he has found to be effective. Hemophiliacs are alert to what they feel to be mismanagement of their condition by medical personnel and frequently feel they know more about their own requirements than do some physicians.

Pain is caused, generally, by internal bleeding which may cause intense suffering. Hemarthropathies are caused by repeated bleeding into the joints and can result in severe limitation of movement and use of limbs. Although the majority of the respondents reported the presence of arthropathies, most also reported that they had received no rehabilitative care for their crippling. Effective corrective and rehabilitative procedures have been developed by orthopedists and physiatrists, and many respondents could probably benefit from such measures, especially if applied at an early age.

The unpredictability of onset of spontaneous bleeding or of injury which may lead to confinement is another problem. Some respondents said they had been able to achieve an accepting attitude toward this situation, doing what they could when they were well, knowing there would be times of forced inaction. Others found the unpredictability to be a major cause of concern and frustration, interfering with their employment and with making plans of any sort for the near or distant future. Disappointments because of inability to carry out planned and ongoing activities were frequently experienced. At times spontaneous bleeding may even be attributed to excitement or other emotional factors associated with an anticipated activity, such as attendance at school or plans for a holiday.

As would be evident, many hemophiliacs have imminent awareness of the possibility of dying. Many know of hemophilic relatives or acquaintances who have died of hemorrhages. The unpredictability of onset of hemorrhaging poses a constant threat. The feeling exists that one may be perfectly well one day and gravely ill or dead the next. Related are the problems associated with the occurrence of disease or injury, other than hemophilia, where surgery may be required to correct the condition but cannot be performed because of possible complications. Some hemophiliacs have undergone surgery, but the risk is often high so that such procedures are generally avoided. Problems frequently arise around dental care; many hemophiliacs suffer from untreated dental disease causing discomfort as well as detriment to health.

EDUCATIONAL ACHIEVEMENT

A relatively large proportion of hemophiliacs have inadequate educational achievements; however, there are also a sizeable proportion with high educational achievement.

As noted, absenteeism is the major barrier to successful completion of schooling by hemophiliacs. Some of our respondents had never been to school, some had received only tutoring; most, however, had attended regular school. At least 34 percent of the respondents had not completed high school; at least 22 percent had received no high school education. On the other hand, 24 percent had education beyond high school and 11 percent had graduated from college, including 6 percent who attended or completed graduate school.

The main reasons for discontinuing school prematurely were health status and retardation due to absenteeism.

But in addition, some hemophiliacs encountered school policies detrimental to their progress and which indicated a lack of understanding on the part of school personnel. Our respondents generally believed that attendance at a regular school was most beneficial to their personal development, despite such problems as refusal of admission, retardation in grade level because of absence, negative attitudes of teachers regarding their potential, and inappropriateness of school programs and policies in relation to their special requirements.

It is true, of course, that not all hemophiliacs encounter problems either with school policies or with their own performance.

Several special factors seem related to successful school achievement for hemophiliacs. These include a positive attitude on the part of parents, encouraging the boy to participate and to achieve in a non-over protective atmosphere; flexible school policies which take into consideration a high absentee-rate, and which may include provisions for tutoring and other special privileges; the general attitudes and activity level of the hemophilic child–the development of attitudes of participation and self-sufficiency rather than those of passivity-dependency with an emphasis on disability. Familial overprotection and the discouraging experiences of confinement due to hemorrhaging and other barriers to participation and activity are probably important factors in attitude development. Severity of hemophilia is not necessarily related to school achievement.

It is also clear that school achievement is highly related to later success.

THE ROLE OF SOCIETY IN THE LIFE OF THE HEMOPHILIAC

This many-faceted topic has great and far-reaching implications for all hemophiliacs; even though we have noted some gradual improvements, in many ways society still presents serious barriers toward the hemophiliac's achieving a successful adaptation and an adequate social role.

The basic social problem is a lack of knowledge about and understanding of hemophiliacs on the part of other members of society.

This problem stems from several sources, including unfamiliarity with the disease, because of the relative infrequency of its occurrence, and lack of information or misinformation to the public. In much public information there is an overemphasis on the disabling effects of hemophilia, and underemphasis on the positive potentials of hemophiliacs. As a result, many hemophiliacs experience stigmatization and discrimination.

Some public misconceptions seem to stem from simple lack of information. A large segment of the public have never heard of hemophilia and most of those who have, hold only vague notions. Our respondents believe that the misinformed public reaction is often a blend of pity for the victims and aversion to the condition. Underlying the aversion is fear that hemophiliacs are in danger of bleeding to death from the slightest cut. That internal bleeding is a far more real problem is virtually unknown.

It is likely that a *considerable number of hemophiliacs are unknown to various agencies such as hemophilia associations, and to medical facilities such as hospitals and clinics.* One possible indication of this is found in the racial bias in our own study. Among undetected hemophiliacs may be those who have such slight bleeding tendencies that they require no, or very little, special medical attention.

While the present number of hemophiliacs is small, *it is likely that the incidence of hemophilia will increase as more hemophiliacs survive to reproductive age.*

The public image of the hemophiliac is not only vague and distorted, but importantly it also impedes successful social adaptation as an adult.

The hemophiliac is set apart from the rest of society. He is seen as special, fragile, "living on (other persons') blood,"(19), and incapable of leading a "normal" life. Of necessity, there is a perceived social distance between him and others in his society. One of the effects of lifelong perception of difference can be seen in the tendency to conceal the condition.

It is not unusual for hemophiliacs to conceal their condition, especially from employers. This behavior was fairly common among respondents and might be found to exist even more widely if the entire population of hemophiliacs were sampled.

Employers often will not hire hemophiliacs. At least 50 percent of our respondents had been turned down by employers for jobs because of hemophilia, often repeatedly. Concealment of hemophilia from the employer was resorted to in order to avoid such rejection. In some such cases, the hemophiliac may experience no more problems than the nonhemophilic worker. Often, however, there are problems of maintaining the deception, the hemophiliac is forced to invent plausible reasons for absences from work. These problems, in turn, occasion anxiety for the hemophiliac and often loss of his job. According to the respondents, the reasons for being turned down for employment were unrealistic ones; this was one reason why they resorted to dissembling.

Hemophiliacs are often held back from job advancement by employers. Some respondents had been discharged when the employer learned of their hemophilia; some had been lowered in status and pay, although the respondents felt they had been performing adequately on the job. Many had been refused advancement.

Insurance companies and Workmen's Compensation policies are often cited by employers in refusing to hire hemophiliacs. The employer may feel that hemophiliacs present an extraordinary liability risk and will not hire them for that reason, even though the hemophiliac may offer to sign a waiver of liability in the event of injury. A few of our respondents had been permitted to sign such a waiver and were hired; one respondent said it had been necessary for him to agree to forego full retirement benefits.

Hemophiliacs feel that employers have an erroneous understanding of their condition and work potential. Most hemophiliacs feel capable of adequate, sometimes superior, performance in their vocations. In general, however, employers are of the opinion that hemophiliacs are so severely handicapped that they have poor employment potential.

The benefits of medical and life insurance are often denied the hemophiliac. Hemophiliacs feel that the reasons for refusal are based on a lack of understanding of their condition along with exagerated views of their disability on the part of insurance companies.

Access to formal education has been denied some hemophiliacs on the basis of disability. Some schools as well as universities have refused to admit hemophiliacs because of liability risk and the opinion that they are especially handicapped.

The generally held view or the hemophiliac as severely disabled may influence the attitudes and expectations of some hemophiliacs regarding their own potential. Some hemophiliacs seem to have accepted the idea that hemophiliacs are too handicapped to participate effectively in a normal social role, and live their lives according to this belief. It is not surprising to find that some members of this population, as well as the parents of hemophiliac children, have assimilated the attitudes of society.

While it might be expected that hemophiliacs often require

some form of financial aid, we found that *only a small number of the respondents were recipients of social security and disability payments, public assistance from state vocational rehabilitation agencies.* Some respondents had been refused assistance by the various agencies. Some had been offered assistance which had proved to be impractical for them or not adapted to their needs. Some respondents found that agency personnel had little understanding or acquaintance with hemophilia.

The most important reason for sparse receipt of public aid may be that hemophiliacs and their families do not know where to find it. They may desire to receive vocational training or assistance in finding jobs, but are unaware of their frequent eligibility for the public programs in these fields.

There is evidence, also, that welfare and rehabilitation agencies have unclear policies regarding services to hemophiliacs, probably because of the relative infrequency of their contacts. The potential of hemophiliacs as members of the working force appears to be poorly understood, and the kinds of vocational training offered to them are usually limited to those appropriate to the severely handicapped.

RECOMMENDATIONS

The recommendations to follow have to some extent been implied in the conclusions. The two conclusions which have the most relevance are those first and last discussed: that most hemophiliacs are capable of the normally expected role performance of an adult male in society; and that the prevalent public image that the hemophiliac is too handicapped to do so militates against his satisfactory life-adjustment in many important ways.

More Available Information About Hemophilia

Communication to the public regarding hemophilia should be increased and improved in order to widen general understanding of the physical aspects of the disease and to present a more realistic picture of the hemophiliac than merely emphasizing his disability.

Public education could serve to increase the number of blood donors as well as to decrease public stigmatization and avoidance. It could be beneficial in increasing employers' willingness to hire hemophiliacs. Educators and other professional workers need to increase their understanding of the potentialities of hemophiliacs in educational and vocational achievement.

Reevaluation and Extension of Rehabilitation Efforts

The contacts of hemophiliacs with welfare agencies in general and with rehabilitation agencies in particular have been inadequate. Such contacts should be increased through planned measures in childhood and young adulthood in order to provide assistance and guidance toward general adjustment and vocational achievement. Vocational rehabilitation workers can enhance their ability to work with this group by greater familiarity with the problems of hemophiliacs and with the many occupations hemophiliacs can engage in. From such familiarity, recognition will grow that absenteeism rather than disability or the presence of physical hazard is the major occupational handicap.

Vocational Counseling

Hemophiliacs tend to grow up under circumstances imposing upon them many isolating differences. They sometimes do not play with children in a normal fashion. In view of this tendency toward isolation and consequent complications in establishing normal roles, early vocational counseling is of utmost importance. Hemophiliacs should be counseled and trained for jobs suitable to their capacities, in which not only their work needs are met and at which they can make a living, but also their needs for social contacts can be gratified. In this respect the tendency to teach isolating occupations such as watch repair to hemophilia patients is a serious error. Watch repairing is an occupation that is usually carried on in near seclusion and in a very confined space; both of these aspects are physically and psychologically bad for many hemophiliacs.

Early Detection and Action Regarding Adjustment Problems

Since life patterns and self-concept are established early in family, peer, and social interactions, it is important to provide for (1) early detection of problems, individual and group counseling for parents, family members, and hemophiliacs and (2) special alertness to school performance, attendance, and activity level, so that remedial measures can be taken and performance and activity maximized.

Parent Counseling

Every parent of a hemophilic child has to deal with an uncertainty problem. By being active and participating normally with his peers, a child may become injured and thereby subject to severe physical risk. A child who is protected from such participation can become a social cripple. Where to draw the line between protection and participation is an area in which we have little precise knowledge. Parents of hemophiliacs, with their natural emotional involvements, often cannot make this decision on their own. They run a great risk of guilt feelings, no matter what happens, either for being too overprotective or for not being protective enough. Physicians and other professionals are in a better position to discuss these risks and can make clear to parents that there is no set answer to the uncertainty problem. No one can guarantee that a child will not injure himself, no matter now protected, and no one can assure parents that by being protective they will not create a problem perhaps worse than the physical problems at risk.

Active participation in play and goal-oriented pursuits, development of self-sufficiency and self-confidence should be encouraged as goals of parent counseling programs.

Life-Adjustment Counseling

Complex life-adjustment problems can be predicted to occur with every hemophilic patient. Since their occurrence is a certainty, the absence of specialized counseling services for adults as well as parents indicates that there is a gap between what is technically possible and actually realized.

Continuously available professional counseling for hemophilic adults in their problems of social adjustment is essential and can contribute importantly to vocational achievement.

Genetic Counseling

Hemophilia is a hereditary disorder, the pattern of genetic transmission of which is well understood. In view of this fact, genetic counseling can proceed far more definitely and with more certainty than is true in other hereditary conditions. Such counseling is needed not only for the patient, but for his entire family, and particularly the female relatives. The absence of such a program in most areas, the unavailability of specialists to provide such counseling even when it is sought, should be looked at on a national basis.

It would be useful for genetic counselors in hemophilia to have knowledge of the varying attitudes and defense mechanisms used by hemophiliacs and their families. Unless they have this kind of information, counselors will not be able to work effectively. Counseling of this nature not only involves knowledge of the genetic patterns of the disorder, which are fairly simple, but also understanding of the psychology of the patients and the defense mechanisms that are likely to be employed.

Disability Insurance

Job opportunities for hemophiliacs are reduced by the fact that in most jobs, employees must be covered by disability insurance. Such insurance usually cannot be written for hemophiliacs because actuarial risks are too high. It is not reasonable to expect employers to assume such an added risk. If hemophiliacs have a bleeding episode, they may be away from work for days, weeks, and even months. Therefore, if hemophiliacs are to be more widely and stably employed, provisions have to be made to exempt them from disability insurance or to provide a subsidized national insurance program which will cover their medical needs, irrespective of who employs them. This would give employers an incentive for hiring hemophiliacs. It would relieve them from having to assume the medical risks which must be carried for other employees.

Preplanned Care

Hemophilia patients are now given treatment in larger cities, well-equipped hospitals, and special clinics that often cooperate with the Hemophilia Foundations. Smaller communities and rural areas lack such specialized centers. It is therefore reasonable to assume that many hemophilia patients suffer and some die unnecessarily because the provision of medical facilities falls short of technical knowledge.

Hemophilia is not a disorder of such medical magnitude that, like mental disorder or tuberculosis, it would require a very expensive national or state-supported program of care, although the treatment costs are nearly always beyond the income of families with hemophilic members. The absence of a well-planned, preventively oriented care program has serious consequences. Hemophilia is a disorder where the failure to treat early and decisively increases the frequency of severe impairments. For example, many state vocational rehabilitation agencies are interested in aiding hemophilia patients but usually see them too late, when there is already an impairment. If the nature of the disease were better understood and a comprehensive program of community care existed, the vocational rehabilitation services could begin before impairment and work on a preventive basis. This would mean getting to the children and their parents with a planned program of physical care and psychosocial counseling, through the cooperation of State Crippled Children's, vocational rehabilitation, and other public and private agencies.

Such a preventive approach might also reduce the overall costs of care. At the present time, medical care of hemophilic patients is very expensive because of the frequency of illness and disability. A preventive program that would make it less necessary to provide preventable physical rehabilitation would in all likelihood save money over the long run.

AN EPILOGUE

THIS book has tried to present the contemporary situation of the hemophiliac from the standpoint of current behavioral science knowledge and research. Inevitably, though, the scientific analyst is an "outsider;" his "objectivity," while useful in some ways, imposes barriers for the reader in capturing the essence, the realities of life-experience.

After the manuscript was completed, the writer came across a self-report by one of our respondents that eloquently sums up these realities, perhaps more so than many pages of scientific, objective analysis.

We produce this statement as an epilogue, a summary of this book's message, believing that readers will join us in thanking its anonymous author for "telling it like it is."

Alfred H. Katz

"First of all, no kid likes to go to a doctor. I wonder why! To this day I very seldom call mine, or go to the hospital. Why? I think it's a throw-back to when I was a tot. I remember a cut done for a transfusion when I was a tot. I was more frightened. But I probably thought he was "killing" me. Here is a beef that I still carry to this day. Why can't the doctors, nurses, parents treat kids more like humans? Don't they think we don't know or will understand? Why can't they explain? I remember waking up and seeing a strange man looking at me. He was a doctor my folks called. When you're young it scares you. Or you're laying in bed and doctors come in to look at you—strangers. And a group of student doctors come in or student nurses. Why in hell don't they ask first? These people ask questions, prod, and look at you. It's not so bad now that I'm older, but when a kid is 10 to 15 he ought to know the score of the show, if he is one of the characters. I think that a doctor should confide in a patient. It makes better relations and understandings. Kids are human, not cattle to be ignored; so why doesn't the doctor talk to them instead of brushing their questions aside with—"this will make you better."

To this day, doctors give me the impression that they are top-man when dealing with me. But when you get right down to it, they are working for me. The doctor does his job and I pay him. Just like any business. Many times I know what is wrong, and don't need him to confirm it. You know that being a bleeder is quite expensive and I can't afford a doctor *every* time I start bleeding.

I don't know about other hemophiliacs, but being a bleeder is like leading 2 lives or duo personality. When I'm "well" I'm on the go all the time. I go out dancing and dating, and work when I can—just like the Joneses. Occasionally, booze it up with the boys. But when I get hemorrhaging, when it puts me in bed or the house, my life changes. I don't see many people. I don't call or invite many in. I guess I don't feel well at times. But even so, I don't go out unless I'm in the mood. My interests vary or I lose interest when I get "laid up", or what interested me when I was sick doesn't interest me when I'm well. I even think differently. It is probably that many don't know that I'm a bleeder. Some reasons—I don't want people to know—and, I don't give a damn either who knows it, that I'm a bleeder at other times. It depends on what I think or choose to do at the time.

It is hard to tell a kid that he shouldn't do this or that, and you can't be babied. I imagine there are some who are worse off than me. But he should try everything. So he fails! Try again! If it is doing him harm, try moving to something. Everybody can't do everything. A hemophiliac can hurt an elbow in a bathtub, or playing ball. You may as well do it at something you like doing. (Anyway, what boy likes to take a bath rather than play ball?) I have heard where many hemophiliacs are overprotected. If he doesn't get hurt bodily, he'll only get hurt in other ways with being afraid and frustrated. I have played baseball, touch football plus other ball games. I remember playing tackle football once. I kicked and threw the football, not as far as the other boys, but I threw it and kicked it just the same.

The doctors told me to get rid of my bicycle. It would injure the knee more. I don't believe they (specialists) sat down to talk to me. They didn't tell me, or my parents didn't tell me just what the doctors said. A bicycle to a 12 year old—how do you think that just by telling him to get rid of his new bicycle that he would? Well, I didn't get rid of it. Maybe their reasons came true, or I would have hurt the knee other ways and times. The places I've been with that bicycle I could have never have walked to. Many times I couldn't walk but the bike got me home. How would I have gotten to the meadows to shoot my BB gun with the other boys? I shot my share of enemies in war games. I probably felt I could have won WW II single handed.

To this day, I dance to rock'roll or jitter-bug. I have been in a crowded dance floor and not gotten hurt. Then, I've been on a floor where there was hardly anyone else and gotten hurt. I've been kicked, stepped on, and crushed, and have never felt better. Then, there are times when I do "feel it." I wish to state that I'm not on a black leather jacket kick. But I do like dancing and have a good time when I do. If I don't feel so "hot" I just take it easy, so I won't miss work. I just do what I've a mind to do, but take it easy.

About three years ago I started playing the guitar by ear. I always wanted to play an instrument, but I held back when I was a kid. You know, shy, scared, not used to other kids, maybe I'd hold the instrument wrong when I had a sore arm, or inferior feeling. So now I play a guitar. At times the arms and wrists get sore. But what bothers me is my sensitive finger tips. I can't get a decent callous. I think nothing hurts as much as the ears of the family as I sit a-pickin' and a-singin'. I'm no Elvis, but I can bang the hell out of the guitar.

Maybe all this will catch up to me some day. If I think about it, though, I expect it will. But I always said, "I'm going to keep going until I can go no more." Right or wrong.

P.S. It seems to me that so much of my life has been wasted. There is so much that I may have done or attempted if I had money, proper training and education. The mind is young, but the body feels years older. (I.N. Hemophiliac Age: 25.)

REFERENCES

1. AGLE, D.P., and MATTSON, AKE: Psychiatric and Social Care of Patients with Hereditary Hemorrhagic Disease. Study supported by the National Hemophilia Foundation (Northern Ohio Chapter), National Institutes of Health, Public Health Service.
2. BAHNSON, CLAUS: Psychosomatic Aspects of Hemophilia. Paper read at the 9th International Conference for Prophylactic Medicine and Social Hygiene, Mitterrcloy, Aust., Sept., 1966.
3. BIGGS, R., and MacFARLAND, R.G.: Treatment of Haemophilia and Other Coagulation Disorders. Oxford, England, Blackwell Scientific Publications, 1966.
4. BRONKS, I.G., and BLACKBURN, E.K.: Socio-medical study of hemophilia and related states. Brit J Prev Soc Med, (No.2,Apr), 1968.
5. CONNOR, FRANCES P.: Education of the child with hemophilia. Proc Inst Hemophilia, Oct 22-3, 1964, June 10-11, 1965, The National Hemophilia Foundation, New York, p.66.
6. FORREST, TESS: The Paternal roots of male character development. Psychoanal Rev, 54:54, 1967.
7. IBID., p. 55.
8. IBID, p. 56.
9. IBID., p. 57.
10. FUNKE, G.N., and PATTON, D.D.: Epidemiology of Hemophilia. Unpublished paper (written May, 1956). UCLA Medical Center, Los Angeles, Calif.
11. GINZBERG, ELI M.: Manpower in a Service Economy, in Training Health Service Workers: The Critical Challenge. Washington, U.S. Dept. of Labor, 1966.
12. KATZ, ALFRED H.: Social adaptation in chronic illness: a study of hemophilia. Amer J Public Health, 53:1670-71.
13. KATZ, ALFRED H.: Some psychosocial problems in hemophilia. Social Casework, June, 1959.
14. KATZ, ALFRED H., and GOLDY, FLORENCE B.: Social adaptation in hemophilia. Children, Sept-Oct, 1963, pp. 189-93.
15. KERR, C.B.: The management of Haemophilia, Australasian Medical Publishing Co., 1962.
16. MASSIE, ROBERT: They Live on Borrowed Blood. Saturday Evening Post, May 4, 1963, pp. 31-34.
17. MATTSON, AKE, and GROSS, SAMUEL: Adaptational and Defensive Behavior in Young Hemophiliacs and Their Parents. National Hemophilia Foundation (Northern Ohio Chapter), (mimeographed, 18 pp., 1966.)
18. PARSONS, T., and BALES, R.F.: Family, Socialization and Interaction Process. New York, Free Press, 1955.
19. RUSALEM, HERBERT: Problems in the Vocational Development of the Hemophilic Individual. Paper presented at 3rd International Hemophilia Symposium, Montreal, Aug. 1968.

20. SALZMAN, E.W., and BRITTEN, A.: Hemorrhage and Thrombosis. Boston, Little, Brown and Co., 1965.
21. Study of the Psychosocial Antecedents to Hemorrhages in Hemophilic Patients. Project Report #RD-1597-P, Dept of Psychiatry, Jefferson Medical College, Philadelphia, June, 1967.
22. U.S. Census of Population 1960. U.S. Dept of Commerce, Bureau of the Census.

INDEX